New Senior's Diabetic

Cookbook for Beginners

2000+ Days of Easy, Tasty & Low-Carb Recipes You Love to Master Pre-Diabetes and Type 2 Diabetes with Ease| 6-Week Meal Plan for a Healthy Lifestyle

Annie H. Hawk

TABLE OF
CONTENTS

Introduction

Welcome to the New Senior's Diabetic Cookbook for Beginners, a culinary compass designed to guide you through the dietary maze of diabetes. In these pages, we embark on a journey to redefine your cooking experience in the face of diabetes. Aging gracefully doesn't mean surrendering to the whims of diabetes; it means embracing food as a source of joy and vitality rather than a series of limitations.

But this cookbook is more than just a collection of recipes – it's a comprehensive guide to living well with diabetes. Alongside our delicious dishes, you'll find practical tips, helpful advice, and valuable insights to help you navigate the challenges of managing your condition. From understanding the basics of diabetes to mastering meal planning and portion control, we're here to support you every step of the way.

Over time, as I shared my diabetic-friendly recipes with friends, family, and online communities, I witnessed the positive impact they had on individuals living with diabetes. From helping to stabilize blood sugar levels to promoting overall health and vitality, these recipes became a source of empowerment and hope for many. Let's embark on this culinary adventure together and discover the joy of cooking without limits!

Understanding Diabetes

Diabetes is a chronic metabolic disorder characterised by elevated blood glucose levels. Over the years, there have been significant changes in the understanding and management of diabetes.

In the late 19th and early 20th centuries, researchers made key discoveries, including the identification of the pancreas as the site of insulin production and the isolation of insulin in 1921 by Frederick Banting, Charles Best and John McLeod. This groundbreaking discovery marked a turning point in the management of diabetes, transforming it from a fatal disease to a manageable chronic condition.

Since then, our understanding of diabetes has continued to evolve, driven by advancements in medical research, technology, and public health initiatives. The classification of diabetes into type 1, type 2, gestational, and other forms has enabled tailored approaches to treatment and management. Moreover, the discovery of additional hormones and signaling pathways involved in glucose metabolism has provided insights into the complex interplay of factors contributing to diabetes development and progression.

In recent decades, the focus has shifted from simply managing blood glucose levels to addressing the multifaceted aspects of diabetes care, including prevention, lifestyle modification, and holistic patient-centered approaches. Emerging technologies such as continuous glucose monitoring (CGM) systems, insulin pumps, and telemedicine platforms have revolutionized diabetes management, offering greater convenience, precision, and real-time insights for patients and healthcare providers alike.

Furthermore, the recognition of diabetes as a global public health crisis has spurred concerted efforts to raise awareness, improve access to care, and implement population-wide interventions to curb the rising prevalence of diabetes and its associated complications. From community-based education programs to policy initiatives promoting healthier environments and food systems, a comprehensive approach is essential to tackling the multifactorial nature of diabetes.

Current State of Diabetes

Diabetes is a prevalent health problem across the globe, so it is vital to understand its current status. With the prevalence of diabetes on the rise globally. Studying the current trends, challenges and advances in diabetes management is essential for developing effective prevention and treatment strategies.

Classification: Current understanding of diabetes recognizes various types, including type 1, type 2, gestational diabetes, and other less common forms. Each type has distinct etiologies, risk factors, and management strategies, allowing for tailored approaches to treatment and care.

Pathophysiology: Advances in research have elucidated the underlying mechanisms involved in diabetes development and progression. This includes

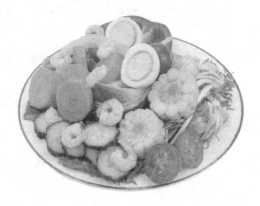

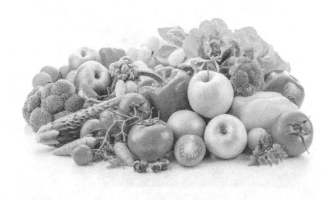

the role of insulin resistance, beta-cell dysfunction, autoimmune processes, genetic predisposition, and environmental factors, providing insights into potential targets for therapeutic interventions.

Complications: Improved understanding of the long-term complications associated with diabetes, such as cardiovascular disease, neuropathy, nephropathy, and retinopathy, has highlighted the importance of early detection and aggressive management to prevent or delay adverse outcomes.

Lifestyle Factors: Recognizing the significant impact of lifestyle factors, such as diet, physical activity, stress, and sleep, on diabetes management has led to greater emphasis on holistic approaches to care. Lifestyle interventions, including dietary modifications, exercise programs, and behavioral therapies, play a central role in diabetes prevention and management.

Technological Innovations: The integration of technology, such as continuous glucose monitoring systems, insulin pumps, and mobile health applications, has revolutionized diabetes management. These tools provide real-time data, facilitate self-management, and empower individuals with diabetes to make informed decisions about their health, thereby improving outcomes and quality of life.

The several types of diabetes

Diabetes is a chronic condition characterized by high levels of glucose (sugar) in the blood. There are three main types of diabetes:

Type 1 Diabetes: This autoimmune disease occurs when the immune system mistakenly attacks and destroys the insulin-producing cells in the pancreas. As a result, the body cannot produce insulin, leading to high blood sugar levels. Type 1 diabetes typically develops in childhood or adolescence, and individuals with this type of diabetes require insulin therapy for life.

Type 2 Diabetes: Type 2 diabetes is the most common form of diabetes, accounting for around 90% of cases worldwide. It occurs when the body becomes resistant to insulin or does not produce enough insulin to maintain normal blood sugar levels. Type 2 diabetes is often linked to lifestyle factors such as obesity, physical inactivity, and poor diet. It can usually be managed through lifestyle changes, medication, and sometimes insulin therapy.

Gestational Diabetes: This type of diabetes occurs during pregnancy and is characterized by high blood sugar levels that develop or are first recognized during pregnancy. Gestational diabetes increases the risk of complications during pregnancy and childbirth for both the mother and the baby. While gestational diabetes typically resolves after giving birth, women who have had gestational diabetes are at increased risk of developing type 2 diabetes later in life.

How to control diabetes through diet and lifestyle

Controlling diabetes through diet and lifestyle is essential for managing blood sugar levels and preventing complications. By making healthy food choices and incorporating regular physical activity into daily routines, individuals with diabetes can improve their overall health and well-being. Understanding the role of nutrition and lifestyle factors is key to achieving optimal diabetes management.

Balanced Diet: Adopting a balanced diet rich in whole grains, fruits, vegetables, lean proteins, and healthy fats is essential for controlling diabetes. Focus on controlling portion sizes and monitoring carbohydrate intake to manage blood sugar levels effectively.

Regular Physical Activity: Incorporating regular exercise into your routine can help improve insulin sensitivity and lower blood sugar levels. Aim for at least 150 minutes of moderate-intensity aerobic activity per week, along with strength training exercises to build muscle and improve overall health.

Monitoring Blood Sugar Levels: Regular monitoring of blood sugar levels is crucial for diabetes

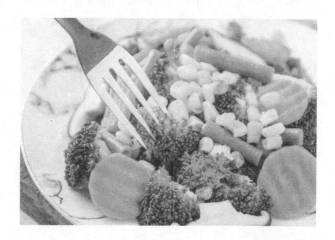

management. Use a glucometer to check blood sugar levels as recommended by your healthcare provider and adjust your diet and medication accordingly to maintain stable blood sugar levels.

Stress Management and Sleep: Chronic stress and inadequate sleep can negatively impact blood sugar levels and overall health. Practice stress-reducing techniques such as mindfulness, meditation, or deep breathing exercises, and aim for 7-9 hours of quality sleep each night to support diabetes management.

Foods to avoid for diabetics

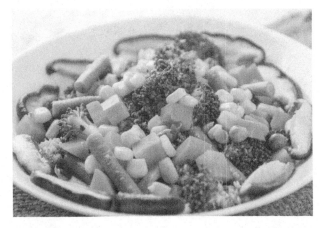

Understanding which foods to avoid is crucial for individuals managing diabetes, as certain foods can cause spikes in blood sugar levels. By identifying and avoiding these foods, individuals can better regulate their blood sugar and reduce the risk of complications associated with diabetes.

Sugary Foods: Avoid consuming sugary snacks, candies, desserts, and sweetened beverages, as they can cause rapid spikes in blood sugar levels.

Refined Carbohydrates: Limit intake of refined carbohydrates like white bread, white rice, and pasta, which can lead to elevated blood sugar levels.

Processed Foods: Stay away from processed foods high in unhealthy fats, sodium, and added sugars, such as fast food, packaged snacks, and pre-packaged meals.

Saturated and Trans Fats: Minimize consumption of foods rich in saturated and trans fats, including fried foods, fatty cuts of meat, and commercially baked goods, as they can increase the risk of heart disease and insulin resistance.

High-Sodium Foods: Reduce intake of high-sodium foods like canned soups, processed meats, and salty snacks, as they can contribute to high blood pressure and other complications associated with diabetes.

Foods to be consumed by diabetics

Choosing the right foods is essential for individuals with diabetes to help manage blood sugar levels and

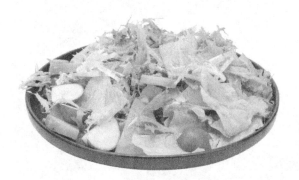

maintain overall health. By focusing on nutrient-dense, low-glycemic foods such as vegetables, fruits, whole grains, lean proteins, and healthy fats, individuals can better control their diabetes and improve their quality of life.

Non-Starchy Vegetables: Incorporate a variety of non-starchy vegetables such as leafy greens, broccoli, cauliflower, and peppers, as they are low in carbohydrates and calories but rich in vitamins, minerals, and fiber.

Whole Grains: Choose whole grains like brown rice, quinoa, oats, and whole wheat bread over refined grains, as they provide more fiber and nutrients and have a lower glycemic index, helping to regulate blood sugar levels.

Lean Proteins: Opt for lean protein sources such as skinless poultry, fish, tofu, legumes, and eggs, as they can help stabilize blood sugar levels and promote satiety without causing spikes in insulin.

Healthy Fats: Include sources of healthy fats like avocados, nuts, seeds, and olive oil in your diet, as they can improve insulin sensitivity, reduce inflammation, and support heart health.

Low-Glycemic Fruits: Enjoy fruits such as berries, apples, citrus fruits, and melons in moderation, as they are lower in sugar and have a lower glycemic index compared to tropical fruits and dried fruits.

Dairy Products: Choose low-fat or non-fat dairy products like yogurt, milk, and cheese as sources of calcium and protein, but be mindful of added sugars in flavored varieties.

Herbs and Spices: Use herbs and spices like cinnamon, turmeric, ginger, and garlic to add flavor to your meals without adding extra calories or carbohydrates, and some may even have beneficial effects on blood sugar control.

Water: Stay hydrated by drinking plenty of water throughout the day, as it helps regulate blood sugar levels, supports kidney function, and promotes overall health.

Designed to help you meet your dietary needs

without compromising on taste or enjoyment, this cookbook is your comprehensive guide to cooking with diabetes.

Whether you're looking for a hearty breakfast, a comforting main course, or a sweet treat, you'll find recipes that satisfy your cravings while keeping you healthy.

Useful tips for switching to a diabetic diet

Transitioning to a diabetic diet can feel overwhelming at first, but with the right approach and guidance, it becomes manageable. Here are some helpful tips to make the switch:

- Educate Yourself: Understanding the principles of a diabetic diet is essential. Learn about carbohydrate counting, glycemic index, portion control, and the importance of balanced meals. Knowledge empowers you to make informed food choices.
- Consult a Registered Dietitian: They can help you create a meal plan, navigate food labels, and address any questions or concerns you have about your diet.
- Spread Out Carbohydrates: Distribute your carbohydrate intake evenly throughout the day to prevent spikes and dips in blood sugar levels. Aim for balanced meals and snacks that contain a combination of carbohydrates, protein, and healthy fats.
- Stay Hydrated: Drink plenty of water throughout the day to stay hydrated and support healthy blood sugar levels. Limit sugary drinks and alcohol, which can cause blood sugar spikes and contribute to dehydration.
- Be Mindful of Fat and Sodium: Choose sources of unsaturated fats such as avocados, nuts, seeds, and olive oil. Additionally, watch your sodium intake and opt for low-sodium or salt-free options when possible to support heart health.
- Plan and Prep Meals: Planning and preparing meals in advance can help you stay on track with your diabetic diet, especially during busy times. Set aside time each week to plan your meals, create a shopping list, and batch cook healthy recipes that you can enjoy throughout the week. Having nutritious meals and snacks readily available reduces the temptation to reach for unhealthy options when hunger strikes.
- Stay Consistent: Consistency is key when managing diabetes through diet. Aim to eat regular meals and snacks at consistent times each day to help stabilize blood sugar levels and prevent fluctuations.
- Stay Motivated: Staying motivated and committed to your diabetic diet can be challenging at times, especially when faced with temptation or setbacks. Find sources of motivation that resonate with you, whether it's achieving better health, improving energy levels, or reducing medication dependence. Celebrate your successes and remind yourself of your goals to stay focused on your journey.

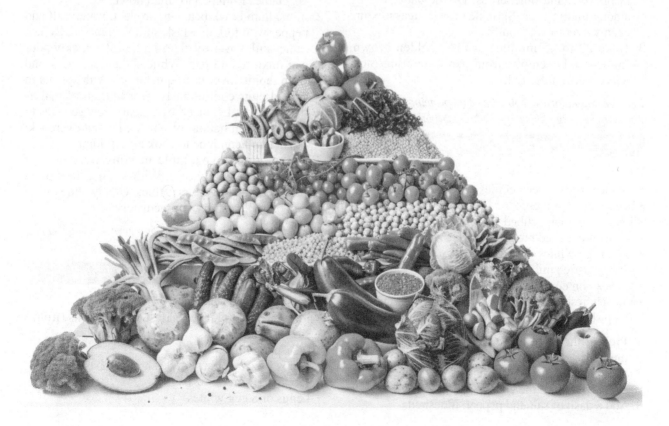

Chapter 1 Breakfasts

Double-Berry Muffins

Prep time: 15 minutes / Cook time: 20 to 25 minutes / Makes 12 muffins

- ¼ cup packed brown sugar
- ½ teaspoon ground cinnamon
- 1 cup fat-free (skim) milk
- ¼ cup unsweetened applesauce
- 2 tablespoons canola oil
- ½ teaspoon vanilla
- 1 egg or ¼ cup fat-free egg product
- 2 cups all-purpose flour
- ⅓ cup granulated sugar
- 3 teaspoons baking powder
- ½ teaspoon salt
- ½ cup fresh or frozen (thawed and drained) raspberries
- ½ cup fresh or frozen (thawed and drained) blueberries

1. Heat oven to 400°F. Place paper baking cup in each of 12 regular-size muffin cups, or grease bottoms only with shortening. In small bowl, mix brown sugar and cinnamon; set aside.
2. In large bowl, beat milk, applesauce, oil, vanilla and egg with fork or whisk. Stir in flour, granulated sugar, baking powder and salt all at once just until flour is moistened (batter will be lumpy). Fold in raspberries and blueberries. Divide batter evenly among muffin cups. Sprinkle brown sugar mixture evenly over tops of muffins.
3. Bake 20 to 25 minutes or until golden brown. Immediately remove from pan to cooling rack. Serve warm if desired.

Per Serving:calories: 160 / fat: 3g / protein: 3g / carbs: 30g / sugars: 12g / fiber: 1g / sodium: 240mg

Mini Breakfast Quiches

Prep time: 10 minutes / Cook time: 20 minutes / Serves 6

- 4 ounces diced green chilies
- ¼ cup diced pimiento
- 1 small eggplant, cubed
- 3 cups precooked brown rice
- ½ cup egg whites
- ⅓ cup fat-free milk
- ½ teaspoon cumin
- 1 bunch fresh cilantro or Italian parsley, finely chopped
- 1 cup shredded reduced-fat cheddar cheese, divided

1. Preheat the oven to 400 degrees. Spray a 12-cup muffin tin with nonstick cooking spray.
2. In a large mixing bowl, combine all the ingredients except ½ cup of the cheese.
3. Add a dash of salt and pepper, if desired.

4. Spoon the mixture evenly into muffin cups, and sprinkle with the remaining cheese. Bake for 12–15 minutes or until set. Carefully remove the quiches from the pan, arrange on a platter, and serve.

Per Serving:calories: 189 / fat: 3g / protein: 11g / carbs: 31g / sugars: 6g / fiber: 5g / sodium: 214mg

Veggie-Stuffed Omelet

Prep time: 15 minutes / Cook time: 10 minutes / Serves 1

- 1 teaspoon olive or canola oil
- 2 tablespoons chopped red bell pepper
- 1 tablespoon chopped onion
- ¼ cup sliced fresh mushrooms
- 1 cup loosely packed fresh baby spinach leaves, rinsed
- ½ cup fat-free egg product or 2 eggs, beaten
- 1 tablespoon water
- Pinch salt
- Pinch pepper
- 1 tablespoon shredded reduced-fat Cheddar cheese

1. In 8-inch nonstick skillet, heat oil over medium-high heat. Add bell pepper, onion and mushrooms to oil. Cook 2 minutes, stirring frequently, until onion is tender. Stir in spinach; continue cooking and stirring just until spinach wilts. Transfer vegetables from pan to small bowl.
2. In medium bowl, beat egg product, water, salt and pepper with fork or whisk until well mixed. Reheat same skillet over medium-high heat. Quickly pour egg mixture into pan. While sliding pan back and forth rapidly over heat, quickly stir with spatula to spread eggs continuously over bottom of pan as they thicken. Let stand over heat a few seconds to lightly brown bottom of omelet. Do not overcook; omelet will continue to cook after folding.
3. Place cooked vegetable mixture over half of omelet; top with cheese. With spatula, fold other half of omelet over vegetables. Gently slide out of pan onto plate. Serve immediately.

Per Serving:calorie: 140 / fat: 5g / protein: 16g / carbs: 6g / sugars: 3g / fiber: 2g / sodium: 470mg

Potato, Egg and Sausage Frittata

Prep time: 30 minutes / Cook time: 20 minutes / Serves 4

- 4 frozen soy-protein breakfast sausage links (from 8-oz box), thawed
- 1 teaspoon olive oil
- 2 cups frozen country-style shredded hash brown potatoes (from 30-oz bag)
- 4 eggs or 8 egg whites

- 1/4 cup fat-free (skim) milk
- 1/4 teaspoon salt
- 1/8 teaspoon dried basil leaves
- 1/8 teaspoon dried oregano leaves
- 1 1/2 cups chopped plum (Roma) tomatoes
- 1/2 cup shredded mozzarella and Asiago cheese blend with garlic (2 oz)
- Pepper, if desired
- Chopped green onion, if desired

1. Cut each sausage link into 8 pieces. Coat 10-inch nonstick skillet with oil; heat over medium heat. Add sausage and potatoes; cook 6 to 8 minutes, stirring occasionally, until potatoes are golden brown.
2. In small bowl, beat eggs and milk with fork or whisk until well blended. Pour egg mixture over potato mixture. Cook uncovered over medium-low heat about 5 minutes; as mixture begins to set on bottom and side, gently lift cooked portions with spatula so that thin, uncooked portion can flow to bottom. Cook until eggs are thickened throughout but still moist; avoid constant stirring.
3. Sprinkle salt, basil, oregano, tomatoes and cheese over eggs. Reduce heat to low; cover and cook about 5 minutes or until center is set and cheese is melted. Sprinkle with pepper and green onion.

Per Serving:calorie: 280 / fat: 12g / protein: 17g / carbs: 26g / sugars: 5g / fiber: 3g / sodium: 590mg

Shakshuka

Prep time: 5 minutes / Cook time: 25 minutes / Serves 4

- 2 tablespoons extra-virgin olive oil
- 1 onion, diced
- 2 tablespoons tomato paste
- 2 red bell peppers, diced
- 2 tablespoons harissa (optional)
- 4 garlic cloves, minced
- 2 teaspoons ground cumin
- 1/2 teaspoon ground coriander (optional)
- 1 teaspoon smoked paprika
- 2 (14-ounce) cans diced tomatoes
- 4 large eggs
- 1/2 cup plain Greek yogurt
- Bread, for dipping (optional)

1. Heat the extra-virgin olive oil in a Dutch oven or large saucepan over medium heat. When it starts to shimmer, add the onion and cook until translucent, about 3 minutes.
2. Add the tomato paste, peppers, harissa (if using), garlic, cumin, coriander (if using), paprika, and tomatoes. Bring to a simmer and cook 10 to 15 minutes, until the peppers are cooked and the sauce is thick. Adjust the seasoning as desired.
3. Make four wells in the mixture with the back of a large spoon and gently break one egg into each

well. Cover the saucepan and simmer gently until the egg whites are set but the yolks are still runny, 5 to 8 minutes.
4. Remove the saucepan from the heat and spoon the tomato mixture and one cooked egg into each of four bowls. Top with the Greek yogurt and serve with bread (if using).

Per Serving:calories: 229 / fat: 13g / protein: 11g / carbs: 20g / sugars: 13g / fiber: 7g / sodium: 127mg

Avocado and Goat Cheese Toast

Prep time: 5 minutes / Cook time: 0 minutes / Serves 2

- 2 slices whole-wheat thin-sliced bread (I love Ezekiel sprouted bread and Dave's Killer Bread)
- 1/2 avocado
- 2 tablespoons crumbled goat cheese
- Salt

1. In a toaster or broiler, toast the bread until browned.
2. Remove the flesh from the avocado. In a medium bowl, use a fork to mash the avocado flesh. Spread it onto the toast.
3. Sprinkle with the goat cheese and season lightly with salt.
4. Add any toppings and serve.

Per Serving:calories: 137 / fat: 6g / protein: 5g / carbs: 18g / sugars: 0g / fiber: 5g / sodium: 195mg

Homemade Turkey Breakfast Sausage

Prep time: 10 minutes / Cook time: 10 minutes / Serves 8

- 1 pound lean ground turkey
- 1/2 teaspoon salt
- 1/2 teaspoon dried sage
- 1/2 teaspoon dried thyme
- 1/2 teaspoon freshly ground black pepper
- 1/4 teaspoon ground fennel seeds
- 1 teaspoon extra-virgin olive oil

1. In a large mixing bowl, combine the ground turkey, salt, sage, thyme, pepper, and fennel. Mix well.
2. Shape the meat into 8 small, round patties.
3. Heat the olive oil in a skillet over medium-high heat. Cook the patties in the skillet for 3 to 4 minutes on each side until browned and cooked through.
4. Serve warm, or store in an airtight container in the refrigerator for up to 3 days or in the freezer for up to 1 month.

Per Serving:calories: 92/ fat: 5g / protein: 11g / carbs: 0g / sugars: 0g / fiber: 0g / sodium: 156mg

Chorizo Mexican Breakfast Pizzas

Prep time: 15 minutes / Cook time: 15 minutes / Serves 4

- 6 ounces chorizo sausage, casing removed,

crumbled, or 6 ounces bulk chorizo sausage
- 2 (10-inch) whole-grain lower-carb lavash flatbreads or tortillas
- ¼ cup chunky-style salsa
- ½ cup black beans with cumin and chili spices (from 15-ounce can)
- ½ cup chopped tomatoes
- ½ cup frozen whole-kernel corn, thawed
- ¼ cup reduced-fat shredded Cheddar cheese (1 ounce)
- 1 tablespoon chopped fresh cilantro
- 2 teaspoons crumbed cotija (white Mexican) cheese

1. Heat oven to 425°F. In 8-inch skillet, cook sausage over medium heat 4 to 5 minutes or until brown; drain.
2. On 1 large or 2 small cookie sheets, place flatbreads. Spread each with 2 tablespoons salsa. Top each with half the chorizo, beans, tomatoes, corn and Cheddar cheese.
3. Bake about 8 minutes or until cheese is melted. Sprinkle each with half the cilantro and cotija cheese; cut into wedges. Serve immediately.

Per Serving:calories: 330 / fat: 2g / protein: 20g / carbs: 19g / sugars: 2g / fiber: 6g / sodium: 1030mg

Lentil, Squash, and Tomato Omelet

Prep time: 5 minutes / Cook time: 45 minutes / Serves 2

- 1 cup water
- ⅓ cup dried lentils, picked over, rinsed, and drained
- Extra-virgin olive oil cooking spray
- 1 medium zucchini, thinly sliced
- ½ cup grape tomatoes, coarsely chopped
- 1 garlic clove, chopped
- 2 tablespoons chopped fresh chives
- 2 large eggs
- 2 tablespoons nonfat milk

1. Preheat the oven to 350°F.
2. In a small saucepan set over high heat, heat the water until it boils.
3. Add the lentils. Reduce the heat to low. Simmer for about 15 minutes, or until most of the liquid has been absorbed. In a colander, drain and set aside.
4. Lightly coat an 8- or 9-inch nonstick skillet with cooking spray. Place the skillet over medium-high heat.
5. Add the zucchini, tomatoes, garlic, and chives. Sauté for 5 to 10 minutes, stirring frequently, or until soft.
6. Add the lentils to the skillet.
7. In a medium bowl, beat together the eggs and milk with a fork.
8. Lightly coat a small casserole or baking dish with cooking spray.
9. In the bottom of the prepared dish, spread the vegetable mixture.
10. Pour the egg mixture over. Use a fork to distribute evenly.
11. Place the dish in the preheated oven. Bake for 15 to 20 minutes, or until the dish is set in the middle.
12. Slice in half and enjoy!

Per Serving:calories: 209 / fat: 6g / protein: 16g / carbs: 25g / sugars: 4g / fiber: 5g / sodium: 90mg

Baked Berry Coconut Oatmeal

Prep time: 10 minutes / Cook time: 35 minutes / Serves 6

- 2 cups rolled oats
- ¼ cup shredded unsweetened coconut
- 1 teaspoon baking powder
- ½ teaspoon ground cinnamon
- ¼ teaspoon sea salt
- 2 cups skim milk
- ¼ cup melted coconut oil, plus extra for greasing the baking dish
- 1 egg
- 1 teaspoon pure vanilla extract
- 2 cups fresh blueberries
- ⅛ cup chopped pecans, for garnish
- 1 teaspoon chopped fresh mint leaves, for garnish

1. Preheat the oven to 350°F.
2. Lightly oil a 2-quart baking dish and set it aside.
3. In a medium bowl, stir together the oats, coconut, baking powder, cinnamon, and salt.
4. In a small bowl, whisk together the milk, oil, egg, and vanilla until well blended.
5. Layer half the dry ingredients in the baking dish, top with half the berries, then spoon the remaining half of the dry ingredients and the rest of the berries on top.
6. Pour the wet ingredients evenly into the baking dish. Tap it lightly on the counter to disperse the wet ingredients throughout.
7. Bake the casserole, uncovered, until the oats are tender, about 35 minutes.
8. Serve immediately, topped with the pecans and mint.

Per Serving:calories: 253 / fat: 15g / protein: 10g / carbs: 33g / sugars: 10g / fiber: 7g / sodium: 145mg

Pumpkin–Peanut Butter Single-Serve Muffins

Prep time: 10 minutes / Cook time: 25 minutes / Serves 2

- 2 tablespoons powdered peanut butter
- 2 tablespoons coconut flour
- 2 tablespoons finely ground flaxseed
- 1 teaspoon pumpkin pie spice
- ½ teaspoon baking powder
- 1 tablespoon dried cranberries
- ½ cup water
- 1 cup canned pumpkin

- 2 large eggs
- ½ teaspoon vanilla extract
- Extra-virgin olive oil cooking spray

1. Preheat the oven to 350°F.
2. In a medium bowl, stir together the powdered peanut butter, coconut flour, flaxseed, pumpkin pie spice, baking powder, dried cranberries, and water.
3. In a separate medium bowl, whisk together the pumpkin and eggs until smooth.
4. Add the pumpkin mixture to the dry ingredients. Stir to combine.
5. Add the vanilla. Mix together well.
6. Spray 2 (8-ounce) ramekins with cooking spray.
7. Spoon half of the batter into each ramekin.
8. Place the ramekins on a baking and carefully transfer the sheet to the preheated oven. Bake for 25 minutes, or until a toothpick in the center comes out clean. Enjoy immediately!

Per Serving:calories: 286 / fat: 16g / protein: 15g / carbs: 24g / sugars: 9g / fiber: 7g / sodium: 189mg

Cinnamon French Toast

Prep time: 10 minutes / Cook time: 20 minutes / Serves 8

- 3 eggs
- 2 cups low-fat milk
- 2 tablespoons maple syrup
- 15 drops liquid stevia
- 2 teaspoons vanilla extract
- 2 teaspoons cinnamon
- Pinch salt
- 16 ounces whole wheat bread, cubed and left out overnight to go stale
- 1½ cups water

1. In a medium bowl, whisk together the eggs, milk, maple syrup, Stevia, vanilla, cinnamon, and salt. Stir in the cubes of whole wheat bread.
2. You will need a 7-inch round baking pan for this. Spray the inside with nonstick spray, then pour the bread mixture into the pan.
3. Place the trivet in the bottom of the inner pot, then pour in the water.
4. Make foil sling and insert it onto the trivet. Carefully place the 7-inch pan on top of the foil sling/trivet.
5. Secure the lid to the locked position, then make sure the vent is turned to sealing.
6. Press the Manual button and use the "+/-" button to set the Instant Pot for 20 minutes.
7. When cook time is up, let the Instant Pot release naturally for 5 minutes, then quick release the rest

Per Serving:calories: 75 / fat: 3g / protein: 4g / carbs: 7g / sugars: 6g / fiber: 0g / sodium: 74mg

Blueberry Cornmeal Muffins

Prep time: 5 minutes / Cook time: 25 minutes / Makes 12 muffins

- 2 cups oat flour
- ½ cup fine corn flour
- ¼ cup coconut sugar
- 2 teaspoons baking powder
- ½ teaspoon baking soda
- ¼ teaspoon sea salt
- 1 teaspoon lemon zest
- ½ cup + 2 to 3 tablespoons plain nondairy yogurt
- ¼ cup pure maple syrup
- ½ cup plain low-fat nondairy milk
- 1 teaspoon lemon juice or apple cider vinegar
- 1 cup frozen or fresh blueberries
- 1 tablespoon oat flour

1. Preheat the oven to 350°F. Line a muffin pan with 12 parchment cupcake liners.
2. In a large bowl, combine the oat flour, corn flour, sugar, baking powder, baking soda, salt, and lemon zest. Stir well. In a medium bowl, combine the yogurt, syrup, milk, and lemon juice or apple cider vinegar, and stir to combine. Add the wet ingredients to the dry and mix until just combined. Toss the berries with the oat flour, and fold them into the batter. Spoon the batter into the muffin liners. Bake for 25 minutes. Remove from the oven and let the muffins cool in the pan for a couple of minutes, then transfer to a cooling rack.

Per Serving:calorie: 152 / fat: 2g / protein: 4g / carbs: 31g / sugars: 11g / fiber: 3g / sodium: 191mg

Bacon and Tomato Frittata

Prep time: 20 minutes / Cook time: 12 minutes / Serves 4

- 1 carton (16 ounces) fat-free egg product
- ¼ teaspoon salt-free garlic-and-herb seasoning
- 2 teaspoons canola oil
- 4 medium green onions, sliced (¼ cup)
- ½ cup sliced celery
- 2 large plum (Roma) tomatoes, sliced
- ¼ cup shredded sharp reduced-fat Cheddar cheese (2 ounces)
- 2 tablespoons real bacon pieces (from 2. 8 ounces package)
- 2 tablespoons light sour cream, if desired

1. In medium bowl, mix egg product and garlic-and-herb seasoning; set aside.
2. In 10-inch nonstick ovenproof skillet, heat oil over medium heat. Add onions and celery; cook and stir 1 minute. Reduce heat to medium-low. Pour in egg mixture. Cook 6 to 9 minutes, gently lifting edges of cooked portions with spatula so that uncooked egg mixture can flow to bottom of skillet, until set.

3. Set oven control to broil. Top frittata with tomatoes, cheese and bacon. Broil with top 4 inches from heat 1 to 2 minutes or until cheese is melted. Top each serving with sour cream.

Per Serving:calories: 110 / fat: 4g / protein: 15g / carbs: 4g / sugars: 2g / fiber: 1g / sodium: 400mg

Baked Eggs

Prep time: 15 minutes / Cook time: 20 minutes / Serves 8

- 1 cup water
- 2 tablespoons no-trans-fat tub margarine, melted
- 1 cup reduced-fat buttermilk baking mix
- 1½ cups fat-free cottage cheese
- 2 teaspoons chopped onion
- 1 teaspoon dried parsley
- ½ cup grated reduced-fat cheddar cheese
- 1 egg, slightly beaten
- 1¼ cups egg substitute
- 1 cup fat-free milk

1. Place the steaming rack into the bottom of the inner pot and pour in 1 cup of water.
2. Grease a round springform pan that will fit into the inner pot of the Instant Pot.
3. Pour melted margarine into springform pan.
4. Mix together buttermilk baking mix, cottage cheese, onion, parsley, cheese, egg, egg substitute, and milk in large mixing bowl.
5. Pour mixture over melted margarine. Stir slightly to distribute margarine.
6. Place the springform pan onto the steaming rack, close the lid, and secure to the locking position. Be sure the vent is turned to sealing. Set for 20 minutes on Manual at high pressure.
7. Let the pressure release naturally.
8. Carefully remove the springform pan with the handles of the steaming rack and allow to stand 10 minutes before cutting and serving.

Per Serving:calories: 155 / fat: 5g / protein: 12g / carbs: 15g / sugars: 4g / fiber: 0g / sodium: 460mg

Cheesy Scrambled Eggs

Prep time: 2 minutes / Cook time: 9 minutes / Serves 2

- 1 teaspoon unsalted butter
- 2 large eggs
- 2 tablespoons milk
- 2 tablespoons shredded Cheddar cheese
- Salt and freshly ground black pepper, to taste

1. Preheat the air fryer to 300°F (149°C). Place the butter in a baking pan and cook for 1 to 2 minutes, until melted.
2. In a small bowl, whisk together the eggs, milk, and cheese. Season with salt and black pepper. Transfer the mixture to the pan.

3. Cook for 3 minutes. Stir the eggs and push them toward the center of the pan.
4. Cook for another 2 minutes, then stir again. Cook for another 2 minutes, until the eggs are just cooked. Serve warm.

Per Serving:calories: 122 / fat: 9g / protein: 9g / carbs: 1g / sugars: 1g / fiber: 0g / sodium: 357mg

Hoe Cakes

Prep time: 10 minutes / Cook time: 15 minutes / Makes 16 to 18

- 1 medium egg
- ½ cup fat-free milk
- 2 cups cornmeal
- 3 teaspoons baking powder
- 1 tablespoon unsalted non-hydrogenated plant-based butter, for greasing the pan

1. In a medium bowl, whisk the egg and milk together.
2. In a separate medium bowl, whisk the cornmeal and baking powder together.
3. Fold the dry ingredients into the wet ingredients until incorporated.
4. In a skillet, melt the butter over medium heat.
5. Add the batter in ¼-cup dollops to the pan (no more than 4 dollops at a time, spaced 1 to 2 inches apart).
6. When the edges become golden brown, turn the cakes, and cook for 30 to 60 seconds more. Repeat until no batter remains.

Per Serving:calories: 85 / fat: 1g / protein: 2g / carbs: 16g / sugars: 1g / fiber: 1g / sodium: 10mg

Stovetop Granola

Prep time: 10 minutes / Cook time: 10 minutes / Makes 4½ cups

- 1½ cups grains (rolled oats, rye flakes, or any flaked grain)
- ¼ cup vegetable, grapeseed, or extra-virgin olive oil
- ¼ cup honey or maple syrup
- 1 tablespoon spice (cinnamon, chai spices, turmeric, ginger, or cloves)
- 1 tablespoon citrus zest (orange, lemon, lime, or grapefruit) (optional)
- 1¼ cups roasted, chopped nuts (almonds, walnuts, or pistachios)
- ¾ cup seeds (sunflower, pumpkin, sesame, hemp, ground chia, or ground flaxseed)
- ½ cup dried fruit (golden raisins, apricots, raisins, dates, figs, or cranberries)
- Kosher salt

1. Heat a large dry skillet, preferably cast iron, over medium-high heat. Add the grains and cook,

stirring frequently, until golden brown and toasty. Remove the grains from the skillet and transfer them to a small bowl.
2. Reduce the heat to medium, return the skillet to the heat, and add the vegetable oil, honey, and spice. Stir until thoroughly combined and bring to a simmer.
3. Once the mixture begins to bubble, reduce the heat to low and add the citrus zest (if using), toasted grains, nuts, seeds, and dried fruit. Stir and cook for another 2 minutes or until the granola is sticky and you can smell the spices. Adjust the seasonings as desired and add salt to taste.
4. Allow the granola to cool before storing it in an airtight container at room temperature for up to 6 months.

Per Serving: *calories: 259 / fat: 13g / protein: 6g / carbs: 35g / sugars: 10g / fiber: 6g / sodium: 4mg*

Quinoa Breakfast Bake with Pistachios and Plums

Prep time: 10 minutes / Cook time: 1 hour / Serves 2

- Extra-virgin olive oil cooking spray
- ⅓ cup dry quinoa, thoroughly rinsed
- 1 teaspoon vanilla extract
- 1 teaspoon cinnamon
- ½ teaspoon nutmeg
- Stevia, for sweetening
- 2 large egg whites
- 1 cup nonfat milk
- 2 plums, chopped, divided
- 4 tablespoons chopped unsalted pistachios, divided

1. Preheat the oven to 350°F.
2. Spray two mini loaf pans with cooking spray. Set aside.
3. In a medium bowl, stir together the quinoa, vanilla, cinnamon, nutmeg, and stevia until the quinoa is coated with the spices.
4. Pour half of the quinoa mixture into each loaf pan.
5. In the same medium bowl, beat the egg whites and thoroughly whisk in the milk.
6. Evenly scatter half of the plums and 2 tablespoons of pistachios in each pan.
7. Pour half of the egg mixture over each loaf. Stir lightly to partially submerge the plums.
8. Place the pans in the preheated oven. Bake for 1 hour, or until the loaves are set, with only a small amount of liquid remaining.
9. Remove from the pans and enjoy hot!

Per Serving: *calories: 295 / fat: 9g / protein: 16g / carbs: 38g / sugars: 14g / fiber: 5g / sodium: 122mg*

Two-Cheese Grits

Prep time: 10 minutes / Cook time: 10 to 12 minutes / Serves 4

- ⅔ cup instant grits
- 1 teaspoon salt

- 1 teaspoon freshly ground black pepper
- ¾ cup milk, whole or 2%
- 1 large egg, beaten
- 3 ounces (85 g) cream cheese, at room temperature
- 1 tablespoon butter, melted
- 1 cup shredded mild Cheddar cheese
- 1 to 2 tablespoons oil

1. In a large bowl, combine the grits, salt, and pepper. Stir in the milk, egg, cream cheese, and butter until blended. Stir in the Cheddar cheese.
2. Preheat the air fryer to 400°F (204°C). Spritz a baking pan with oil.
3. Pour the grits mixture into the prepared pan and place it in the air fryer basket.
4. Cook for 5 minutes. Stir the mixture and cook for 5 minutes more for soupy grits or 7 minutes more for firmer grits.

Per Serving: *calories: 302 / fat: 18g / protein: 13g / carbs: 21g / sugars: 4g / fiber: 1g / sodium: 621mg*

Potato-Bacon Gratin

Prep time: 20 minutes / Cook time: 40 minutes / Serves 8

- 1 tablespoon olive oil
- 6 ounces bag fresh spinach
- 1 clove garlic, minced
- 4 large potatoes, peeled or unpeeled, divided
- 6 ounces Canadian bacon slices, divided
- 5 ounces reduced-fat grated Swiss cheddar, divided
- 1 cup lower-sodium, lower-fat chicken broth

1. Set the Instant Pot to Sauté and pour in the olive oil. Cook the spinach and garlic in olive oil just until spinach is wilted (5 minutes or less). Turn off the instant pot.
2. Cut potatoes into thin slices about ¼" thick.
3. In a springform pan that will fit into the inner pot of your Instant Pot, spray it with nonstick spray then layer ⅓ the potatoes, half the bacon, ⅓ the cheese, and half the wilted spinach.
4. Repeat layers ending with potatoes. Reserve ⅓ cheese for later.
5. Pour chicken broth over all.
6. Wipe the bottom of your Instant Pot to soak up any remaining oil, then add in 2 cups of water and the steaming rack. Place the springform pan on top.
7. Close the lid and secure to the locking position. Be sure the vent is turned to sealing. Set for 35 minutes on Manual at high pressure.
8. Perform a quick release.
9. Top with the remaining cheese, then allow to stand 10 minutes before removing from the Instant Pot, cutting and serving.

Per Serving: *calories: 220 / fat: 7g / protein: 14g / carbs: 28g / sugars: 2g / fiber: 3g / sodium: 415mg*

Bunless Breakfast Turkey Burgers

Prep time: 5 minutes / Cook time: 15 minutes / Serves 4

- 1 pound (454 g) ground turkey breakfast sausage
- ½ teaspoon salt
- ¼ teaspoon ground black pepper
- ¼ cup seeded and chopped green bell pepper
- 2 tablespoons mayonnaise
- 1 medium avocado, peeled, pitted, and sliced

1. In a large bowl, mix sausage with salt, black pepper, bell pepper, and mayonnaise. Form meat into four patties.
2. Place patties into ungreased air fryer basket. Adjust the temperature to 370ºF (188ºC) and air fry for 15 minutes, turning patties halfway through cooking. Burgers will be done when dark brown and they have an internal temperature of at least 165ºF (74ºC).
3. Serve burgers topped with avocado slices on four medium plates.

Per Serving: calories: 283 / fat: 18g / protein: 23g / carbs: 6g / sugars: 1g / fiber: 4g / sodium: 620mg

Sweet Quinoa Cereal

Prep time: 5 minutes / Cook time: 20 minutes / Serves 4

- 1 cup water
- 1 cup skim milk
- 1 cup uncooked quinoa, well rinsed
- ½ teaspoon ground cinnamon
- Pinch sea salt
- 2 tablespoons granulated sweetener
- 1 teaspoon pure vanilla extract
- ¼ cup toasted chopped almonds
- ½ cup sliced strawberries

1. Put the water, milk, quinoa, cinnamon, and salt in a medium saucepan over medium-high heat.
2. Bring the mixture to a boil, then reduce the heat to low.
3. Simmer the quinoa cereal until most of the liquid is gone, about 15 minutes.
4. Remove the cereal from the heat and stir in the sweetener and vanilla.
5. Spoon the cereal into four bowls and top with the almonds and strawberries.

Per Serving: calories: 243 / fat: 6g / protein: 9g / carbs: 39g / sugars: 9g / fiber: 4g / sodium: 30mg

Carrot Pear Smoothie

Prep time: 10 minutes / Cook time: 0 minutes / Serves 2

- 2 carrots, peeled and grated
- 1 ripe pear, unpeeled, cored and chopped
- 2 teaspoons grated fresh ginger
- Juice and zest of 1 lime
- 1 cup water
- ½ teaspoon ground cinnamon
- ¼ teaspoon ground nutmeg

1. Put the carrots, pear, ginger, lime juice, lime zest, water, cinnamon, and nutmeg in a blender and blend until smooth.
2. Pour into two glasses and serve.

Per Serving: calories: 61 / fat: 0g / protein: 1g / carbs: 15g / sugars: 7g / fiber: 4g / sodium: 45mg

Breakfast Hash

Prep time: 10 minutes / Cook time: 30 minutes / Serves 6

- Oil, for spraying
- 3 medium russet potatoes, diced
- ½ yellow onion, diced
- 1 green bell pepper, seeded and diced
- 2 tablespoons olive oil
- 2 teaspoons granulated garlic
- 1 teaspoon salt
- ½ teaspoon freshly ground black pepper

1. Line the air fryer basket with parchment and spray lightly with oil.
2. In a large bowl, mix together the potatoes, onion, bell pepper, and olive oil.
3. Add the garlic, salt, and black pepper and stir until evenly coated.
4. Transfer the mixture to the prepared basket.
5. Air fry at 400ºF (204ºC) for 20 to 30 minutes, shaking or stirring every 10 minutes, until browned and crispy. If you spray the potatoes with a little oil each time you stir, they will get even crispier.

Per Serving: calorie: 124 / fat: 4g / protein: 2g / carbs: 21g / sugars: 2g / fiber: 2g / sodium: 390mg

Canadian Bacon and Egg Muffin Cups

Prep time: 5 minutes / Cook time: 20 minutes / Serves 6

- Cooking spray (for greasing)
- 6 large slices Canadian bacon
- 12 large eggs, beaten
- 1 teaspoon Dijon mustard
- ½ teaspoon sea salt
- Dash hot sauce
- 1 cup shredded Swiss cheese

1. Preheat the oven to 350ºF. Spray 6 nonstick muffin cups with cooking spray.
2. Line each cup with 1 slice of Canadian bacon.
3. In a bowl, whisk together the eggs, mustard, salt, and hot sauce. Fold in the cheese. Spoon the mixture into the muffin cups.
4. Bake until the eggs set, about 20 minutes.

Per Serving: calories: 232 / fat: 15g / protein: 21g / carbs: 2g / sugars: 1g / fiber: 0g / sodium: 498mg

Cottage Cheese Almond Pancakes

Prep time: 10 minutes / Cook time: 20 minutes / Serves 4

- 2 cups low-fat cottage cheese
- 4 egg whites
- 2 eggs
- 1 tablespoon pure vanilla extract
- 1½ cups almond flour
- Nonstick cooking spray

1. Place the cottage cheese, egg whites, eggs, and vanilla in a blender and pulse to combine.
2. Add the almond flour to the blender and blend until smooth.
3. Place a large nonstick skillet over medium heat and lightly coat it with cooking spray.
4. Spoon ¼ cup of batter per pancake, 4 at a time, into the skillet. Cook the pancakes until the bottoms are firm and golden, about 4 minutes.
5. Flip the pancakes over and cook the other side until they are cooked through, about 3 minutes.
6. Remove the pancakes to a plate and repeat with the remaining batter.
7. Serve with fresh fruit.

Per Serving: *calories: 441 / fat: 32g / protein: 30g / carbs: 9g / sugars: 3g / fiber: 5g / sodium: 528mg*

Wild Mushroom Frittata

Prep time: 10 minutes / Cook time: 15 minutes / Serves 4

- 8 large eggs
- ½ cup skim milk
- ¼ teaspoon ground nutmeg
- Sea salt
- Freshly ground black pepper
- 2 teaspoons extra-virgin olive oil
- 2 cups sliced wild mushrooms (cremini, oyster, shiitake, portobello, etc.)
- ½ red onion, chopped
- 1 teaspoon minced garlic
- ½ cup goat cheese, crumbled

1. Preheat the broiler.
2. In a medium bowl, whisk together the eggs, milk, and nutmeg until well combined. Season the egg mixture lightly with salt and pepper and set it aside.
3. Place an ovenproof skillet over medium heat and add the oil, coating the bottom completely by tilting the pan.
4. Sauté the mushrooms, onion, and garlic until translucent, about 7 minutes.
5. Pour the egg mixture into the skillet and cook until the bottom of the frittata is set, lifting the edges of the cooked egg to allow the uncooked egg to seep under.
6. Place the skillet under the broiler until the top is set, about 1 minute.
7. Sprinkle the goat cheese on the frittata and broil

until the cheese is melted, about 1 minute more.
8. Remove from the oven. Cut into 4 wedges to serve.

Per Serving: *calories: 258 / fat: 17g / protein: 19g / carbs: 7g / sugars: 3g / fiber: 1g / sodium: 316mg*

Spaghetti Squash Fritters

Prep time: 15 minutes / Cook time: 8 minutes / Serves 4

- 2 cups cooked spaghetti squash
- 2 tablespoons unsalted butter, softened
- 1 large egg
- ¼ cup blanched finely ground almond flour
- 2 stalks green onion, sliced
- ½ teaspoon garlic powder
- 1 teaspoon dried parsley

1. Remove excess moisture from the squash using a cheesecloth or kitchen towel.
2. Mix all ingredients in a large bowl. Form into four patties.
3. Cut a piece of parchment to fit your air fryer basket. Place each patty on the parchment and place into the air fryer basket.
4. Adjust the temperature to 400ºF (204ºC) and set the timer for 8 minutes.
5. Flip the patties halfway through the cooking time. Serve warm.

Per Serving: *calories: 146 / fat: 12g / protein: 4g / carbs: 7g / sugars: 3g / fiber: 2g / sodium: 36mg*

Smoked Salmon and Asparagus Quiche Cups

Prep time: 15 minutes / Cook time: 15 minutes / Serves 2

- Nonstick cooking spray
- 4 asparagus spears, cut into ½-inch pieces
- 2 tablespoons finely chopped onion
- 3 ounces (85 g) smoked salmon (skinless and boneless), chopped
- 3 large eggs
- 2 tablespoons 2% milk
- ¼ teaspoon dried dill
- Pinch ground white pepper

1. Pour 1½ cups of water into the electric pressure cooker and insert a wire rack or trivet.
2. Lightly spray the bottom and sides of the ramekins with nonstick cooking spray. Divide the asparagus, onion, and salmon between the ramekins.
3. In a measuring cup with a spout, whisk together the eggs, milk, dill, and white pepper. Pour half of the egg mixture into each ramekin. Loosely cover the ramekins with aluminum foil.
4. Carefully place the ramekins inside the pot on the rack.
5. Close and lock the lid of the pressure cooker. Set the valve to sealing.
6. Cook on high pressure for 15 minutes.
7. When the cooking is complete, hit Cancel and

quick release the pressure.

8. Once the pin drops, unlock and remove the lid.
9. Carefully remove the ramekins from the pot. Cool, covered, for 5 minutes.
10. Run a small silicone spatula or a knife around the edge of each ramekin. Invert each quiche onto a small plate and serve.

Per Serving:calories: 180 / fat: 9g / protein: 20g / carbs: 3g / sugars: 1g / fiber: 1g / sodium: 646mg

White Bean–Oat Waffles

Prep time: 10 minutes / Cook time: 20 minutes / Serves 2

- 1 large egg white
- 2 tablespoons finely ground flaxseed
- ½ cup water
- ¼ teaspoon salt
- 1 teaspoon vanilla extract
- ½ cup cannellini beans, drained and rinsed
- 1 teaspoon coconut oil
- 1 teaspoon liquid stevia
- ½ cup old-fashioned rolled oats
- Extra-virgin olive oil cooking spray

1. In a blender, combine the egg white, flaxseed, water, salt, vanilla, cannellini beans, coconut oil, and stevia. Blend on high for 90 seconds.
2. Add the oats. Blend for 1 minute more.
3. Preheat the waffle iron. The batter will thicken to the correct consistency while the waffle iron preheats.
4. Spray the heated waffle iron with cooking spray.
5. Add ¾ cup of batter. Close the waffle iron. Cook for 6 to 8 minutes, or until done. Repeated with the remaining batter.
6. Serve hot, with your favorite sugar-free topping.

Per Serving:calories: 294 / fat: 10g / protein: 13g / carbs: 38g / sugars: 4g / fiber: 9g / sodium: 404mg

Mandarin Orange–Millet Breakfast Bowl

Prep time: 5 minutes / Cook time: 30 minutes / Serves 2

- ⅓ cup millet
- 1 cup nonfat milk
- ½ cup water
- ¼ teaspoon cinnamon
- ¼ teaspoon ground cardamom
- 1 teaspoon vanilla extract
- Pinch salt
- Stevia, for sweetening
- ½ cup canned mandarin oranges, drained
- 2 tablespoons sliced almonds

1. In a small saucepan set over medium-high heat, stir together the millet, milk, water, cinnamon, cardamom, vanilla, salt, and stevia. Bring to a boil. Reduce the heat to low. Cover and simmer for 25 minutes, without stirring. If the liquid is not completely absorbed, cook for 3 to 5 minutes longer, partially covered.
2. Stir in the oranges. Remove from the heat.
3. Top with the sliced almonds and serve.

Per Serving:calories: 254 / fat: 7g / protein: 10g / carbs: 38g / sugars: 12g / fiber: 5g / sodium: 73mg

Mexican Breakfast Pepper Rings

Prep time: 5 minutes / Cook time: 10 minutes / Serves 4

- Olive oil
- 1 large red, yellow, or orange bell pepper, cut into four ¾-inch rings
- 4 eggs
- Salt and freshly ground black pepper, to taste
- 2 teaspoons salsa

1. Preheat the air fryer to 350ºF (177ºC). Lightly spray a baking pan with olive oil.
2. Place 2 bell pepper rings on the pan. Crack one egg into each bell pepper ring. Season with salt and black pepper.
3. Spoon ½ teaspoon of salsa on top of each egg.
4. Place the pan in the air fryer basket. Air fry until the yolk is slightly runny, 5 to 6 minutes or until the yolk is fully cooked, 8 to 10 minutes.
5. Repeat with the remaining 2 pepper rings. Serve hot.

Per Serving:calorie: 93 / fat: 7g / protein: 6g / carbs: 2g / sugars: 1g / fiber: 1g / sodium: 164mg

Summer Veggie Scramble

Prep time: 10 minutes / Cook time: 10 minutes / Serves 4

- 1 teaspoon extra-virgin olive oil
- 1 scallion, white and green parts, finely chopped
- ½ yellow bell pepper, seeded and chopped
- ½ zucchini, diced
- 8 large eggs, beaten
- 1 tomato, cored, seeded, and diced
- 2 teaspoons chopped fresh oregano
- Sea salt
- Freshly ground black pepper

1. Place a large skillet over medium heat and add the olive oil.
2. Add the scallion, bell pepper, and zucchini to the skillet and sauté for about 5 minutes.
3. Pour in the eggs and, using a wooden spoon or spatula, scramble them until thick, firm curds form and the eggs are cooked through, about 5 minutes.
4. Add the tomato and oregano to the skillet and stir to incorporate.
5. Serve seasoned with salt and pepper.

Per Serving:calories: 170 / fat: 11g / protein: 14g / carbs: 4g / sugars: 1g / fiber: 1g / sodium: 157mg

Chapter 2 Beans and Grains

Southwestern Quinoa Salad

Prep time: 15 minutes / Cook time: 25 minutes / Serves 6

- Salad
- 1 cup uncooked quinoa
- 1 large onion, chopped (1 cup)
- 1½ cups reduced-sodium chicken broth
- 1 cup packed fresh cilantro leaves
- ¼ cup raw unsalted hulled pumpkin seeds (pepitas)
- 2 cloves garlic, sliced
- ⅛ teaspoon ground cumin
- 2 tablespoons chopped green chiles (from 4. 5-oz can)
- 1 tablespoon olive oil
- 1 can (15 ounces) no-salt-added black beans, drained, rinsed
- 6 medium plum (Roma) tomatoes, chopped (2 cups)
- 2 tablespoons lime juice
- Garnish
- 1 avocado, pitted, peeled, thinly sliced
- 4 small cilantro sprigs

1. Rinse quinoa thoroughly by placing in a fine-mesh strainer and holding under cold running water until water runs clear; drain well.
2. Spray 3-quart saucepan with cooking spray. Heat over medium heat. Add onion to pan; cook 6 to 8 minutes, stirring occasionally, until golden brown. Stir in quinoa and chicken broth. Heat to boiling; reduce heat. Cover and simmer 10 to 15 minutes or until all liquid is absorbed; remove from heat.
3. Meanwhile, in small food processor, place cilantro, pumpkin seeds, garlic and cumin. Cover; process 5 to 10 seconds, using quick on-and-off motions; scrape side. Add chiles and oil. Cover; process, using quick on-and-off motions, until paste forms.
4. To cooked quinoa, add pesto mixture and the remaining salad ingredients. Refrigerate at least 30 minutes to blend flavors.
5. To serve, divide salad evenly among 4 plates; top each serving with 3 or 4 slices avocado and 1 sprig cilantro.

Per Serving:calorie: 310 / fat: 12g / protein: 13g / carbs: 38g / sugars: 5g / fiber: 9g / sodium: 170mg

Red Beans

Prep time: 10 minutes / Cook time: 45 minutes / Serves 8

- 1 cup crushed tomatoes
- 1 medium yellow onion, chopped
- 2 garlic cloves, minced
- 2 cups dried red kidney beans
- 1 cup roughly chopped green beans
- 4 cups store-bought low-sodium vegetable broth
- 1 teaspoon smoked paprika

1. Select the Sauté setting on an electric pressure cooker, and combine the tomatoes, onion, and garlic. Cook for 3 to 5 minutes, or until softened.
2. Add the kidney beans, green beans, broth, and paprika. Stir to combine.
3. Close and lock the lid, and set the pressure valve to sealing.
4. Change to the Manual/Pressure Cook setting, and cook for 35 minutes.
5. Once cooking is complete, quick-release the pressure. Carefully remove the lid.
6. Serve.

Per Serving:calorie: 73 / fat: 0g / protein: 4g / carbs: 14g / sugars: 4g / fiber: 4g / sodium: 167mg

Coconut-Ginger Rice

Prep time: 10 minutes / Cook time: 20 minutes / Serves 8

- 2½ cups reduced-sodium chicken broth
- ⅔ cup reduced-fat (lite) coconut milk (not cream of coconut)
- 1 tablespoon grated gingerroot
- ½ teaspoon salt
- 1⅓cups uncooked regular long-grain white rice
- 1 teaspoon grated lime peel
- 3 medium green onions, chopped (3 tablespoons)
- 3 tablespoons flaked coconut, toasted*
- Lime slices

1. In 3-quart saucepan, heat broth, coconut milk, gingerroot and salt to boiling over medium-high heat. Stir in rice. Return to boiling. Reduce heat; cover and simmer about 15 minutes or until rice is tender and liquid is absorbed. Remove from heat.
2. Add lime peel and onions; fluff rice mixture lightly with fork to mix. Garnish with coconut and lime slices.

Per Serving:calorie: 150 / fat: 2g / protein: 3g / carbs: 30g / sugars: 1g / fiber: 0g / sodium: 340mg

Sunshine Burgers

Prep time: 10 minutes / Cook time: 18 to 20 minutes / Makes 10 burgers

- 2 cups sliced raw carrots
- 1 large clove garlic, sliced or quartered
- 2 cans (15 ounces each) chickpeas, rinsed and drained
- ¼ cup sliced dry-packed sun-dried tomatoes
- 2 tablespoons tahini
- 1 teaspoon red wine vinegar or apple cider vinegar
- 1 teaspoon smoked paprika
- ½ teaspoon dried rosemary
- ½ teaspoon ground cumin
- ½ teaspoon sea salt

- 1 cup rolled oats

1. In a food processor, combine the carrots and garlic. Pulse several times to mince. Add the chickpeas, tomatoes, tahini, vinegar, paprika, rosemary, cumin, and salt. Puree until well combined, scraping down the sides of the bowl once or twice. Add the oats, and pulse briefly to combine. Refrigerate the mixture for 30 minutes, if possible.
2. Preheat the oven to 400°F. Line a baking sheet with parchment paper.
3. Use an ice cream scoop to scoop the mixture onto the prepared baking sheet, flattening to shape it into patties. Bake for 18 to 20 minutes, flipping the burgers halfway through. Alternatively, you can cook the burgers in a nonstick skillet over medium heat for 6 to 8 minutes Per side, or until golden brown. Serve.

Per Serving:calorie: 137 / fat: 4 / protein: 6g / carbs: 21g / sugars: 4g / fiber: 6g / sodium: 278mg

Stewed Green Beans

Prep time: 5 minutes / Cook time: 10 minutes / Serves 4

- 1 pound green beans, trimmed
- 1 medium tomato, chopped
- ½ yellow onion, chopped
- 1 garlic clove, minced
- 1 teaspoon Creole seasoning
- ¼ cup store-bought low-sodium vegetable broth

1. In an electric pressure cooker, combine the green beans, tomato, onion, garlic, Creole seasoning, and broth.
2. Close and lock the lid, and set the pressure valve to sealing.
3. Select the Manual/Pressure Cook setting, and cook for 10 minutes.
4. Once cooking is complete, quick-release the pressure. Carefully remove the lid.
5. Transfer the beans to a serving dish. Serve warm.

Per Serving:calorie: 58 / fat: 0g / protein: 3g / carbs: 13g / sugars: 7g / fiber: 4g / sodium: 98mg

Colorful Rice Casserole

Prep time: 5 minutes / Cook time: 20 minutes / Serves 12

- 1 tablespoon extra-virgin olive oil
- 1½ pounds zucchini, thinly sliced
- ¾ cup chopped scallions
- 2 cups corn kernels (frozen or fresh; if frozen, defrost)
- One 14. 5-ounce can no-salt-added chopped tomatoes, undrained
- ¼ cup chopped parsley
- 1 teaspoon oregano
- 3 cups cooked brown (or white) rice
- ⅛ teaspoon freshly ground black pepper

1. In a large skillet, heat the oil. Add the zucchini and

scallions, and sauté for 5 minutes.
2. Add the remaining ingredients, cover, reduce heat, and simmer for 10–15 minutes or until the vegetables are heated through. Season with salt, if desired, and pepper. Transfer to a bowl, and serve.

Per Serving:calorie: 109 / fat: 2g / protein: 3g / carbs: 21g / sugars: 4g / fiber: 3g / sodium: 14mg

Sage and Garlic Vegetable Bake

Prep time: 30 minutes / Cook time: 1 hour 15 minutes / Serves 6

- 1 medium butternut squash, peeled, cut into 1-inch pieces (3 cups)
- 2 medium parsnips, peeled, cut into 1-inch pieces (2 cups)
- 2 cans (14. 5 ounces each) stewed tomatoes, undrained
- 2 cups frozen cut green beans
- 1 medium onion, coarsely chopped (½ cup)
- ½ cup uncooked quick-cooking barley
- ½ cup water
- 1 teaspoon dried sage leaves
- ½ teaspoon seasoned salt
- 2 cloves garlic, finely chopped

1. Heat oven to 375°F. In ungreased 3-quart casserole, mix all ingredients, breaking up large pieces of tomatoes.
2. Cover; bake 1 hour to 1 hour 15 minutes or until vegetables and barley are tender.

Per Serving:calorie: 170 / fat: 0g / protein: 4g / carbs: 37g / sugars: 9g / fiber: 8g / sodium: 410mg

Hoppin' John

Prep time: 15 minutes / Cook time: 50 minutes / Serves 12

- 1 tablespoon canola oil
- 2 celery stalks, thinly sliced
- 1 small yellow onion, chopped
- 1 medium green bell pepper, chopped
- 1 tablespoon tomato paste
- 2 garlic cloves, minced
- 2 cups brown rice, rinsed
- 5 cups store-bought low-sodium vegetable broth, divided
- 2 bay leaves
- 1 teaspoon smoked paprika
- 1 teaspoon Creole seasoning
- 1¼ cups frozen black-eyed peas

1. In a Dutch oven, heat the canola oil over medium heat.
2. Add the celery, onion, bell pepper, tomato paste, and garlic and cook, stirring often, for 3 to 5 minutes, or until the vegetables are softened.
3. Add the rice, 4 cups of broth, bay leaves, paprika, and Creole seasoning.
4. Reduce the heat to low, cover, and cook for 30 minutes, or until the rice is tender.

5. Add the black-eyed peas and remaining 1 cup of broth. Mix well, cover, and cook for 12 minutes, or until the peas soften. Discard the bay leaves.
6. Enjoy.

Per Serving:calorie: 155 / fat: 2g / protein: 4g / carbs: 30g / sugars: 1g / fiber: 2g / sodium: 24mg

Italian Bean Burgers

Prep time: 10 minutes / Cook time: 20 minutes / Makes 9 burgers

- 2 cans (14 or 15 ounces each) chickpeas, drained and rinsed
- 1 medium–large clove garlic, cut in half
- 2 tablespoons tomato paste
- 1½ tablespoons red wine vinegar (can substitute apple cider vinegar)
- 1 tablespoon tahini
- 1 teaspoon Dijon mustard
- ½ teaspoon onion powder
- Scant ½ teaspoon sea salt
- 2 tablespoons chopped fresh oregano
- ⅓ cup roughly chopped fresh basil leaves
- 1 cup rolled oats
- ⅓ cup chopped sun-dried tomatoes (not packed in oil)
- ½ cup roughly chopped kalamata or green olives

1. In a food processor, combine the chickpeas, garlic, tomato paste, vinegar, tahini, mustard, onion powder, and salt. Puree until fully combined. Add the oregano, basil, and oats, and pulse briefly. (You want to combine the ingredients but retain some of the basil's texture.) Finally, pulse in the sun-dried tomatoes and olives, again maintaining some texture. Transfer the mixture to a bowl and refrigerate, covered, for 30 minutes or longer.
2. Preheat the oven to 400°F. Line a baking sheet with parchment paper. Use an ice cream scoop to scoop the mixture onto the prepared baking sheet, flattening to shape into patties. Bake for about 20 minutes, flipping the burgers halfway through. Alternatively, you can cook the burgers in a nonstick skillet over medium heat for 6 to 8 minutes Per side, or until golden brown. Serve.

Per Serving:calorie: 148 / fat: 4g / protein: 6g / carbs: 23g / sugars: 4g / fiber: 6g / sodium: 387mg

Rice with Spinach and Feta

Prep time: 10 minutes / Cook time: 15 minutes / Serves 4

- ¾ cup uncooked brown rice
- 1½ cups water
- 1 tablespoon extra-virgin olive oil
- 1 medium onion, diced
- 1 cup sliced mushrooms
- 2 garlic cloves, minced
- 1 tablespoon lemon juice
- ½ teaspoon dried oregano
- 9 cups fresh spinach, stems trimmed, washed, patted dry, and coarsely chopped
- ⅓ cup crumbled fat-free feta cheese
- ⅛ teaspoon freshly ground black pepper

1. In a medium saucepan over medium heat, combine the rice and water. Bring to a boil, cover, reduce heat, and simmer for 15 minutes. Transfer to a serving bowl.
2. In a skillet, heat the oil. Sauté the onion, mushrooms, and garlic for 5 to 7 minutes. Stir in the lemon juice and oregano. Add the spinach, cheese, and pepper, tossing until the spinach is slightly wilted.
3. Toss with rice and serve.

Per Serving:calorie: 205 / fat: 5g / protein: 7g / carbs: 34g / sugars: 2g / fiber: 4g / sodium: 129mg

Quinoa Vegetable Skillet

Prep time: 15 minutes / Cook time: 15 minutes / Serves 6

- 2 cups vegetable broth
- 1 cup quinoa, well rinsed and drained
- 1 teaspoon extra-virgin olive oil
- ½ sweet onion, chopped
- 2 teaspoons minced garlic
- ½ large green zucchini, halved lengthwise and cut into half disks
- 1 red bell pepper, seeded and cut into thin strips
- 1 cup fresh or frozen corn kernels
- 1 teaspoon chopped fresh basil
- Sea salt
- Freshly ground black pepper

1. Place a medium saucepan over medium heat and add the vegetable broth. Bring the broth to a boil and add the quinoa. Cover and reduce the heat to low.
2. Cook until the quinoa has absorbed all the broth, about 15 minutes. Remove from the heat and let it cool slightly.
3. While the quinoa is cooking, place a large skillet over medium-high heat and add the oil.
4. Sauté the onion and garlic until softened and translucent, about 3 minutes.
5. Add the zucchini, bell pepper, and corn, and sauté until the vegetables are tender-crisp, about 5 minutes.
6. Remove the skillet from the heat. Add the cooked quinoa and the basil to the skillet, stirring to combine. Season with salt and pepper, and serve.

Per Serving:calorie: 178 / fat: 2g / protein: 6g / carbs: 35g / sugars: 5g / fiber: 5g / sodium: 375mg

Beet Greens and Black Beans

Prep time: 10 minutes / Cook time: 20 minutes / Serves 4

- 1 tablespoon unsalted non-hydrogenated plant-based butter
- ½ Vidalia onion, thinly sliced

- ½ cup store-bought low-sodium vegetable broth
- 1 bunch beet greens, cut into ribbons
- 1 bunch dandelion greens, cut into ribbons
- 1 (15-ounce) can no-salt-added black beans
- Freshly ground black pepper

1. In a medium skillet, melt the butter over low heat.
2. Add the onion, and sauté for 3 to 5 minutes, or until the onion is translucent.
3. Add the broth and greens. Cover the skillet and cook for 7 to 10 minutes, or until the greens are wilted.
4. Add the black beans and cook for 3 to 5 minutes, or until the beans are tender. Season with black pepper.

Per Serving:calorie: 153 / fat: 3g / protein: 9g / carbs: 25g / sugars: 2g / fiber: 11g / sodium: 312mg

Curried Rice with Pineapple

Prep time: 5 minutes / Cook time: 35 minutes / Serves 8

- 1 onion, chopped
- 1½ cups water
- 1¼ cups low-sodium chicken broth
- 1 cup uncooked brown basmati rice, soaked in water 20 minutes and drained before cooking
- 2 red bell peppers, minced
- 1 teaspoon curry powder
- 1 teaspoon ground turmeric
- 1 teaspoon ground ginger
- 2 garlic cloves, minced
- One 8-ounce can pineapple chunks packed in juice, drained
- ¼ cup sliced almonds, toasted

1. In a medium saucepan, combine the onion, water, and chicken broth. Bring to a boil, and add the rice, peppers, curry powder, turmeric, ginger, and garlic. Cover, placing a paper towel in between the pot and the lid, and reduce the heat. Simmer for 25 minutes.
2. Add the pineapple, and continue to simmer 5–7 minutes more until rice is tender and water is absorbed. Taste and add salt, if desired. Transfer to a serving bowl, and garnish with almonds to serve.

Per Serving:calorie: 144 / fat: 3g / protein: 4g / carbs: 27g / sugars: 6g / fiber: 3g / sodium: 16mg

Barley Squash Risotto

Prep time: 10 minutes / Cook time: 15 minutes / Serves 6

- 1 teaspoon extra-virgin olive oil
- ½ sweet onion, finely chopped
- 1 teaspoon minced garlic
- 2 cups cooked barley
- 2 cups chopped kale
- 2 cups cooked butternut squash, cut into ½-inch cubes
- 2 tablespoons chopped pistachios
- 1 tablespoon chopped fresh thyme
- Sea salt

1. Place a large skillet over medium heat and add the oil.

2. Sauté the onion and garlic until softened and translucent, about 3 minutes.
3. Add the barley and kale, and stir until the grains are heated through and the greens are wilted, about 7 minutes.
4. Stir in the squash, pistachios, and thyme.
5. Cook until the dish is hot, about 4 minutes, and season with salt.

Per Serving:calorie: 158 / fat: 3g / protein: 4g / carbs: 31g / sugars: 3g / fiber: 7g / sodium: 77mg

Edamame-Tabbouleh Salad

Prep time: 20 minutes / Cook time: 10 minutes / Serves 6

- Salad
- 1 package (5. 8 ounces) roasted garlic and olive oil couscous mix
- 1¼ cups water
- 1 teaspoon olive or canola oil
- 1 bag (10 ounces) refrigerated fully cooked ready-to-eat shelled edamame (green soybeans)
- 2 medium tomatoes, seeded, chopped (1½ cups)
- 1 small cucumber, peeled, chopped (1 cup)
- ¼ cup chopped fresh parsley
- Dressing
- 1 teaspoon grated lemon peel
- 2 tablespoons lemon juice
- 1 teaspoon olive or canola oil

1. Make couscous mix as directed on package, using the water and oil.
2. In large bowl, mix couscous and remaining salad ingredients. In small bowl, mix dressing ingredients. Pour dressing over salad; mix well. Serve immediately, or cover and refrigerate until serving time.

Per Serving:calorie: 200 / fat: 5g / protein: 10g / carbs: 28g / sugars: 3g / fiber: 4g / sodium: 270mg

Whole-Wheat Linguine with Kale Pesto

Prep time: 10 minutes / Cook time: 20 minutes / Serves 6

- ½ cup shredded kale
- ½ cup fresh basil
- ½ cup sun-dried tomatoes
- ¼ cup chopped almonds
- 2 tablespoons extra-virgin olive oil
- 8 ounces dry whole-wheat linguine
- ½ cup grated Parmesan cheese

1. Place the kale, basil, sun-dried tomatoes, almonds, and olive oil in a food processor or blender, and pulse until a chunky paste forms, about 2 minutes. Scoop the pesto into a bowl and set it aside.
2. Place a large pot filled with water on high heat and bring to a boil.
3. Cook the pasta al dente, according to the package directions.

4. Drain the pasta and toss it with the pesto and the Parmesan cheese.
5. Serve immediately.

Per Serving:calorie: 365 / fat: 19g / protein: 15g / carbs: 38g / sugars: 3g / fiber: 7g / sodium: 299mg

Sweet Potato Fennel Bake

Prep time: 15 minutes / Cook time: 45 minutes / Serves 4

- 1 teaspoon butter
- 1 fennel bulb, trimmed and thinly sliced
- 2 sweet potatoes, peeled and thinly sliced
- Freshly ground black pepper, to taste
- ½ teaspoon ground cinnamon
- ¼ teaspoon ground nutmeg
- 1 cup low-sodium vegetable broth

1. Preheat the oven to 375°F.
2. Lightly butter a 9-by-11-inch baking dish.
3. Arrange half the fennel in the bottom of the dish and top with half the sweet potatoes.
4. Season the potatoes with black pepper. Sprinkle half the cinnamon and nutmeg on the potatoes.
5. Repeat the layering to use up all the fennel, sweet potatoes, cinnamon, and nutmeg.
6. Pour in the vegetable broth and cover the dish with aluminum foil.
7. Bake until the vegetables are very tender, about 45 minutes.
8. Serve immediately.

Per Serving:calorie: 118 / fat: 1g / protein: 2g / carbs: 28g / sugars: 7g / fiber: 5g / sodium: 127mg

Veggie Unfried Rice

Prep time: 15 minutes / Cook time: 25 minutes / Serves 4

- 1 tablespoon extra-virgin olive oil
- 1 bunch collard greens, stemmed and cut into chiffonade
- ½ cup store-bought low-sodium vegetable broth
- 1 carrot, cut into 2-inch matchsticks
- 1 red onion, thinly sliced
- 1 garlic clove, minced
- 2 tablespoons coconut aminos
- 1 cup cooked brown rice
- 1 large egg
- 1 teaspoon red pepper flakes
- 1 teaspoon paprika

1. In a large Dutch oven, heat the olive oil over medium heat.
2. Add the collard greens and cook for 3 to 5 minutes, or until the greens are wilted.
3. Add the broth, carrot, onion, garlic, and coconut aminos, then cover and cook for 5 to 7 minutes, or until the carrot softens and the onion and garlic are translucent.
4. Uncover, add the rice, and cook for 3 to 5 minutes,

gently mixing all the ingredients together until well combined but not mushy.
5. Crack the egg over the pot and gently scramble the egg. Cook for 2 to 5 minutes, or until the eggs are no longer runny.
6. Remove from the heat and season with the red pepper flakes and paprika.

Per Serving:calorie: 164 / fat: 4g / protein: 9g / carbs: 26g / sugars: 3g / fiber: 9g / sodium: 168mg

Wild Rice with Blueberries and Pumpkin Seeds

Prep time: 15 minutes / Cook time: 45 minutes / Serves 4

- 1 tablespoon extra-virgin olive oil
- ½ sweet onion, chopped
- 2½ cups sodium-free chicken broth
- 1 cup wild rice, rinsed and drained
- Pinch sea salt
- ½ cup toasted pumpkin seeds
- ½ cup blueberries
- 1 teaspoon chopped fresh basil

1. Place a medium saucepan over medium-high heat and add the oil.
2. Sauté the onion until softened and translucent, about 3 minutes.
3. Stir in the broth and bring to a boil.
4. Stir in the rice and salt and reduce the heat to low. Cover and simmer until the rice is tender, about 40 minutes.
5. Drain off any excess broth, if necessary. Stir in the pumpkin seeds, blueberries, and basil.
6. Serve warm.

Per Serving:calorie: 306 / fat: 15g / protein: 12g / carbs: 37g / sugars: 7g / fiber: 6g / sodium: 12mg

Texas Caviar

Prep time: 10 minutes / Cook time: 0 minutes / Serves 6

- 1 cup cooked black-eyed peas
- 1 cup cooked lima beans
- 1 ear fresh corn, kernels removed
- 2 celery stalks, chopped
- 1 red bell pepper, chopped
- ½ red onion, chopped
- 3 tablespoons apple cider vinegar
- 2 tablespoons extra-virgin olive oil
- 1 teaspoon paprika

1. In a large bowl, combine the black-eyed peas, lima beans, corn, celery, bell pepper, and onion.
2. In a small bowl, to make the dressing, whisk the vinegar, oil, and paprika together.
3. Pour the dressing over the bean mixture, and gently mix. Set aside for 15 to 30 minutes, allowing the flavors to come together.

Per Serving:calorie: 142 / fat: 5g / protein: 6g / carbs: 19g / sugars: 3g / fiber: 6g / sodium: 10mg

Chapter 3 Poultry

Fiber-Full Chicken Tostadas

Prep time: 15 minutes / Cook time: 10 minutes / Serves 4

- 1 tablespoon (9 g) chili powder
- ½ tablespoon (5 g) onion powder
- 1 tablespoon (9 g) paprika
- 1 teaspoon garlic powder
- 1 teaspoon ground cumin
- 1 teaspoon dried oregano
- ¼ teaspoon black pepper
- ¼ teaspoon sea salt
- 2 tablespoons (30 ml) cooking oil of choice
- 1 pound (454 g) boneless, skinless chicken breast, cut into 1 to 1½-inch (2. 5 to 3. 8 cm) strips
- 8 corn tostada shells
- 1 (15½ ounces [439 g]) can low-sodium pinto beans, undrained
- 1 cup (30 g) baby arugula leaves, coarsely chopped
- 1 large avocado, peeled and sliced to the desired thickness
- 4 tablespoons (32 g) crumbled queso fresco cheese
- Jalapeño slices (optional)
- Chopped onion (optional)
- Diced tomatoes (optional)

1. In a small bowl, mix together the chili powder, onion powder, paprika, garlic powder, cumin, oregano, black pepper, and sea salt. Add the cooking oil and mix it with the seasonings to make a marinade.
2. Place the chicken strips in a large ziptop plastic bag, then add the marinade. Seal the bag and shake it to coat the chicken with the marinade. (If time permits, marinate the chicken for 30 to 60 minutes.)
3. Heat a large skillet over medium-high heat. Add the chicken strips and cook them for 4 to 5 minutes. Flip the chicken strips and cook them for 3 to 4 minutes, until they are cooked through and no longer pink. Set the skillet aside.
4. Line up the tostada shells on a serving tray. Place the pinto beans in a medium bowl and mash them to the desired consistency. Spread the beans on top of each tostada. Top each tostada with an equal amount of arugula, avocado slices, cheese, chicken and any desired additional toppings, then serve.

Per Serving:*calorie: 547 / fat: 27g / protein: 40g / carbs: 12g / sugars: 1g / fiber: 12g / sodium: 738mg*

Shredded Buffalo Chicken

Prep time: 10 minutes / Cook time: 20 minutes / Serves 8

- 2 tablespoons avocado oil
- ½ cup finely chopped onion
- 1 celery stalk, finely chopped
- 1 large carrot, chopped
- ⅓ cup mild hot sauce (such as Frank's RedHot)
- ½ tablespoon apple cider vinegar
- ¼ teaspoon garlic powder
- 2 bone-in, skin-on chicken breasts (about 2 pounds)

1. Set the electric pressure cooker to the Sauté setting. When the pot is hot, pour in the avocado oil.
2. Sauté the onion, celery, and carrot for 3 to 5 minutes or until the onion begins to soften. Hit Cancel.
3. Stir in the hot sauce, vinegar, and garlic powder. Place the chicken breasts in the sauce, meat-side down.
4. Close and lock the lid of the pressure cooker. Set the valve to sealing.
5. Cook on high pressure for 20 minutes.
6. When cooking is complete, hit Cancel and quick release the pressure. Once the pin drops, unlock and remove the lid.
7. Using tongs, transfer the chicken breasts to a cutting board. When the chicken is cool enough to handle, remove the skin, shred the chicken and return it to the pot. Let the chicken soak in the sauce for at least 5 minutes.
8. Serve immediately.

Per Serving:*calorie: 235 / fat: 14g / protein: 24g / carbs: 2g / sugars: 1g / fiber: 1g / sodium: 142mg*

Kung Pao Chicken and Zucchini Noodles

Prep time: 15 minutes / Cook time: 15 minutes / Serves 2

- For the noodles:
- 2 medium zucchini, ends trimmed
- For the sauce:
- 1½ tablespoons low-sodium soy sauce
- 1 tablespoon balsamic vinegar
- 1 teaspoon hoisin sauce
- 2½ tablespoons water
- 1½ teaspoons red chili paste
- 2 teaspoons granulated stevia
- 2 teaspoons cornstarch
- For the chicken:
- 6 ounces boneless skinless chicken breast, cut into ½-inch pieces
- Salt, to season
- Freshly ground black pepper, to season
- 1 teaspoon extra-virgin olive oil
- 1 teaspoon sesame oil
- 2 garlic cloves, minced
- 1 tablespoon chopped fresh ginger

- ½ red bell pepper, cut into ½-inch pieces
- ½ (8-ounce) can water chestnuts, drained and sliced
- 1 celery stalk, cut into ¾-inch dice
- 2 tablespoons crushed dry-roasted peanuts, divided
- 2 tablespoons scallions, divided

To make the noodles: 1. With a spiralizer or julienne peeler, cut the zucchini lengthwise into spaghetti-like strips. Set aside. To make the sauce: 1. In a small bowl, whisk together the soy sauce, balsamic vinegar, hoisin sauce, water, red chili paste, stevia, and cornstarch. Set aside. To make the chicken: 1. Season the chicken with salt and pepper.

2. In a large, deep nonstick pan or wok set over medium-high heat, heat the olive oil.
3. Add the chicken. Cook for 4 to 5 minutes, stirring, or until browned and cooked through. Transfer the chicken to a plate. Set aside.
4. Return the pan to the stove. Reduce the heat to medium.
5. Add the sesame oil, garlic, and ginger. Cook for about 30 seconds, or until fragrant.
6. Add the red bell pepper, water chestnuts, and celery.
7. Stir in the sauce. Bring to a boil. Reduce the heat to low. Simmer for 1 to 2 minutes, until thick and bubbling.
8. Stir in the zucchini noodles. Cook for about 2 minutes, tossing, until just tender and mixed with the sauce.
9. Add the chicken and any accumulated juices. Stir to combine. Cook for about 2 minutes, or until heated through.
10. Divide the mixture between 2 bowls. Top each serving with 1 tablespoon of peanuts and 1 tablespoon of scallions. Enjoy!

Per Serving:calorie: 322 / fat: 13g / protein: 29g / carbs: 28g / sugars: 12g / fiber: 8g / sodium: 553mg

Easy Chicken Cacciatore

Prep time: 5 minutes / Cook time: 20 minutes / Serves 2

- Extra-virgin olive oil cooking spray
- 1 garlic clove, chopped
- ½ cup chopped red onion
- ¾ cup chopped green bell pepper
- 2 (6-ounce) boneless skinless chicken breasts, cubed
- 1 cup sliced cremini mushrooms
- ½ cup chopped tomatoes, with juice
- 1 cup green beans
- 1 teaspoon dried oregano
- 1 teaspoon dried rosemary

1. Coat a skillet with cooking spray. Place it over medium heat.
2. Add the garlic. Sauté for about 1 minute, or until browned.

3. Add the red onion, green bell pepper, and chicken. Cook for about 6 minutes, or until the chicken is slightly browned, tossing to cook all sides.
4. Stir in the mushrooms, tomatoes, green beans, oregano, and rosemary. Reduce the heat to medium-low. Simmer for 8 to 10 minutes, stirring constantly.
5. Remove from the heat and serve hot.
6. Enjoy!

Per Serving:calorie: 265 / fat: 5g / protein: 42g / carbs: 13g / sugars: 6g / fiber: 4g / sodium: 91mg

Speedy Chicken Cacciatore

Prep time: 5 minutes / Cook time: 30 minutes / Serves 6

- 2 pounds boneless, skinless chicken thighs
- 1½ teaspoons fine sea salt
- ½ teaspoon freshly ground black pepper
- 2 tablespoons extra-virgin olive oil
- 3 garlic cloves, chopped
- 2 large red bell peppers, seeded and cut into ¼ by 2-inch strips
- 2 large yellow onions, sliced
- ½ cup dry red wine
- 1½ teaspoons Italian seasoning
- ½ teaspoon red pepper flakes (optional)
- One 14½ ounces can diced tomatoes and their liquid
- 2 tablespoons tomato paste
- Cooked brown rice or whole-grain pasta for serving

1. Season the chicken thighs on both sides with 1 teaspoon of the salt and the black pepper.
2. Select the Sauté setting on the Instant Pot and heat the oil and garlic for 2 minutes, until the garlic is bubbling but not browned. Add the bell peppers, onions, and remaining ½ teaspoon salt and sauté for 3 minutes, until the onions begin to soften. Stir in the wine, Italian seasoning, and pepper flakes (if using). Using tongs, add the chicken to the pot, turning each piece to coat it in the wine and spices and nestling them in a single layer in the liquid. Pour the tomatoes and their liquid on top of the chicken and dollop the tomato paste on top. Do not stir them in.
3. Secure the lid and set the Pressure Release to Sealing. Press the Cancel button to reset the cooking program, then select the Poultry, Pressure Cook, or Manual setting and set the cooking time for 12 minutes at high pressure. (The pot will take about 15 minutes to come up to pressure before the cooking program begins.)
4. When the cooking program ends, perform a quick pressure release by moving the Pressure Release to Venting, or let the pressure release naturally. Open the pot and, using tongs, transfer the chicken and vegetables to a serving dish.
5. Spoon some of the sauce over the chicken and

serve hot, with the rice on the side.

Per Serving:calories: 297 / fat: 11g / protein: 32g / carbs: 16g / sugars: 3g / fiber: 3g / sodium: 772mg

Herbed Buttermilk Chicken

Prep time: 5 minutes / Cook time: 25 minutes / Serves 4

- 1½ pounds boneless, skinless chicken breasts
- 4 cups buttermilk
- Pinch kosher salt
- Pinch freshly ground black pepper
- 1 cup thinly sliced yellow onion
- 2 tablespoons canola oil
- ¼ cup Italian seasoning
- 1 lemon, cut into wedges

1. In a large bowl or sealable plastic bag, combine the chicken, buttermilk, salt, and pepper. Cover or seal and refrigerate for at least 1 hour and up to 24 hours.
2. When the chicken is ready to cook, preheat the oven to 425°F. Line a baking sheet with parchment paper.
3. Remove the chicken from the buttermilk brine and pat it dry. Place the chicken on the prepared baking sheet along with the onion, and drizzle everything with the canola oil. Toss together on the baking sheet (this will save you a bowl) to coat the chicken and onion evenly.
4. Bake for 25 minutes or until the chicken is cooked through. (If the chicken is thick, you can cut the breasts in half lengthwise. It will cut down on your cook time by half or less. Check the chicken after it's cooked for 8 minutes if the breasts are thin.)
5. Allow the chicken to rest and sprinkle it and the onions with the Italian seasoning.
6. Serve with a squeeze of lemon juice.

Per Serving:calorie: 380 / fat: 14g / protein: 47g / carbs: 16g / sugars: 13g / fiber: 1g / sodium: 543mg

Turkey Stuffed Peppers

Prep time: 15 minutes / Cook time: 50 minutes / Serves 4

- 1 teaspoon extra-virgin olive oil, plus more for greasing the baking dish
- 1 pound ground turkey breast
- ½ sweet onion, chopped
- 1 teaspoon minced garlic
- 1 tomato, diced
- ½ teaspoon chopped fresh basil
- Sea salt
- Freshly ground black pepper
- 4 red bell peppers, tops cut off, seeded
- 2 ounces low-sodium feta cheese

1. Preheat the oven to 350°F.
2. Lightly grease a 9-by-9-inch baking dish with olive oil and set it aside.
3. Place a large skillet over medium heat and add 1

teaspoon of olive oil.
4. Add the turkey to the skillet and cook until it is no longer pink, stirring occasionally to break up the meat and brown it evenly, about 6 minutes.
5. Add the onion and garlic and sauté until softened and translucent, about 3 minutes.
6. Stir in the tomato and basil. Season with salt and pepper.
7. Place the peppers cut-side up in the baking dish. Divide the filling into four equal portions and spoon it into the peppers.
8. Sprinkle the feta cheese on top of the filling.
9. Add ¼ cup of water to the dish and cover with aluminum foil.
10. Bake the peppers until they are soft and heated through, about 40 minutes.

Per Serving:calorie: 285 / fat: 12g / protein: 31g / carbs: 12g / sugars: 8g / fiber: 3g / sodium: 79mg

Spicy Chicken Drumsticks

Prep time: 5 minutes / Cook time: 50 minutes / Serves 2

- ¼ cup plain low-fat yogurt
- 2 tablespoons hot pepper sauce
- Crushed red pepper flakes, to taste
- 4 chicken drumsticks, skinned (about 1 pound)
- ¼ cup dried bread crumbs

1. In a shallow dish, combine the yogurt, hot pepper sauce, and crushed red pepper flakes, mixing well. Add the drumsticks, turning to coat. Cover, and marinate in the refrigerator for 2 to 4 hours.
2. Preheat the oven to 350 degrees.
3. Remove the drumsticks from the marinade, dredge in the bread crumbs, and place in a baking dish. Bake at 350 degrees for 40 to 50 minutes. Transfer to a serving platter, and serve.

Per Serving:calorie: 337 / fat: 10g / protein: 48g / carbs: 12g / sugars: 3g / fiber: 1g / sodium: 501mg

Herb-Roasted Turkey and Vegetables

Prep time: 20 minutes / Cook time: 2 hours / Serves 6

- 2 teaspoons minced garlic
- 1 tablespoon chopped fresh parsley
- 1 teaspoon chopped fresh thyme
- 1 teaspoon chopped fresh rosemary
- 2 pounds boneless, skinless whole turkey breast
- 3 teaspoons extra-virgin olive oil, divided
- Sea salt
- Freshly ground black pepper
- 2 sweet potatoes, peeled and cut into 2-inch chunks
- 2 carrots, peeled and cut into 2-inch chunks
- 2 parsnips, peeled and cut into 2-inch chunks
- 1 sweet onion, peeled and cut into eighths

1. Preheat the oven to 350°F.

2. Line a large roasting pan with aluminum foil and set it aside.
3. In a small bowl, mix together the garlic, parsley, thyme, and rosemary.
4. Place the turkey breast in the roasting pan and rub it all over with 1 teaspoon of olive oil.
5. Rub the garlic-herb mixture all over the turkey and season lightly with salt and pepper.
6. Place the turkey in the oven and roast for 30 minutes.
7. While the turkey is roasting, toss the sweet potatoes, carrots, parsnips, onion, and the remaining 2 teaspoons of olive oil in a large bowl.
8. Remove the turkey from the oven and arrange the vegetables around it.
9. Roast until the turkey is cooked through (170°F internal temperature) and the vegetables are lightly caramelized, about 1 ½ hours.

Per Serving: calorie: 267 / fat: 4g / protein: 35g / carbs: 25g / sugars: 8g / fiber: 5g / sodium: 379mg

Herbed Cornish Hens

Prep time: 5 minutes / Cook time: 30 minutes / Serves 8

• 4 Cornish hens, giblets removed (about 1¼ pound each)
• 2 cups white wine, divided
• 2 garlic cloves, minced
• 1 small onion, minced
• ½ teaspoon celery seeds
• ½ teaspoon poultry seasoning
• ½ teaspoon paprika
• ½ teaspoon dried oregano
• ¼ teaspoon freshly ground black pepper

1. Using a long, sharp knife, split each hen lengthwise. You may also buy precut hens.
2. Place the hens, cavity side up, on a rack in a shallow roasting pan. Pour 1½ cups of the wine over the hens; set aside.
3. In a shallow bowl, combine the garlic, onion, celery seeds, poultry seasoning, paprika, oregano, and pepper. Sprinkle half of the combined seasonings over the cavity of each split half. Cover, and refrigerate. Allow the hens to marinate for 2–3 hours.
4. Preheat the oven to 350 degrees. Bake the hens uncovered for 1 hour. Remove from the oven, turn breast side up, and remove the skin. Pour the remaining ½ cup of wine over the top, and sprinkle with the remaining seasonings.
5. Continue to bake for an additional 25–30 minutes, basting every 10 minutes until the hens are done. Transfer to a serving platter, and serve hot.

Per Serving: calorie: 383 / fat: 10g / protein: 57g / carbs: 3g / sugars: 1g / fiber: 0g / sodium: 197mg

Baked Chicken Stuffed with Collard Greens

Prep time: 10 minutes / Cook time: 30 minutes / Serves 4

• For the gravy
• 2½ cups store-bought low-sodium chicken broth, divided
• 4 tablespoons whole-wheat flour, divided
• 1 medium yellow onion, chopped
• ½ bunch fresh thyme, roughly chopped
• 2 garlic cloves, minced
• 1 bay leaf
• ½ teaspoon celery seeds
• 1 teaspoon Worcestershire sauce
• Freshly ground black pepper
• For the chicken
• 2 boneless, skinless chicken breasts
• Juice of 1 lime
• 1 teaspoon sweet paprika
• ½ teaspoon onion powder
• ½ teaspoon garlic powder
• 2 medium tomatoes, chopped
• 1 bunch collard greens, center stem removed, cut into 1-inch ribbons
• ¼ cup chicken broth (optional)
• Generous pinch red pepper flakes

To make the gravy 1. In a shallow stockpot, combine ½ cup of broth and 1 tablespoon of flour and cook over medium-low heat, whisking until the flour is dissolved. Continue to add 1 cup of broth and the remaining 3 tablespoons of flour in increments until a thick sauce is formed.

2. Add the onion, thyme, garlic, bay leaf, and ½ cup of broth, stirring well. To make the chicken 1. Cut a slit in each chicken breast deep enough for stuffing along its entire length.
2. In a small mixing bowl, massage the chicken all over with the lime juice, paprika, onion powder, and garlic powder.
3. In an electric pressure cooker, combine the tomatoes and collard greens. If the mixture looks dry, add the chicken broth.
4. Close and lock the lid, and set the pressure valve to sealing.
5. Select the Manual/Pressure Cook setting, and cook for 2 minutes.
6. Once cooking is complete, quick-release the pressure. Carefully remove the lid.
7. Using tongs or a slotted spoon, remove the greens while leaving the tomatoes behind.
8. Stuff the chicken breasts with the greens. Lay on the bed of tomatoes in the pressure cooker, with the side with greens facing up.
9. Spoon half of the gravy over the stuffed chicken.
10. Close and lock the lid, and set the pressure valve to sealing.

11. Select the Manual/Pressure Cook setting, and cook for 10 minutes.
12. Once cooking is complete, quick-release the pressure. Carefully remove the lid.
13. Remove the chicken and tomatoes from pressure cooker, and transfer to a serving dish. Season with the red pepper flakes.

Per Serving:calorie: 301 / fat: 6g / protein: 41g / carbs: 24g / sugars: 4g / fiber: 9g / sodium: 155mg

Slow-Roasted Turkey Breast in Beer-Mustard Sauce

Prep time: 5 minutes / Cook time: 2 hour 30 minutes / Serves 10

- 5 pounds, bone-in turkey breast, skin removed
- 1 tablespoon prepared mustard
- ½ cup light beer
- ¼ cup red wine vinegar
- ¾ cup ketchup
- 1 tablespoon no-added-salt tomato paste
- ½ cup spicy no-added-salt tomato juice (or spice up mild juice with several drops of hot pepper sauce)
- ¼ teaspoon freshly ground black pepper

1. Preheat the oven to 350 degrees.
2. Spread the turkey breast with mustard.
3. In a small bowl, combine the beer, vinegar, ketchup, tomato paste, and tomato juice. Pour the mixture over the turkey, and then sprinkle with pepper.
4. Roast, covered, for 1½ hours at 350 degrees. Remove the cover, and roast an additional 1 hour, basting occasionally. Transfer to a serving platter, and serve.

Per Serving:calorie: 280 / fat: 4g / protein: 52g / carbs: 6g / sugars: 4g / fiber: 0g / sodium: 450mg

Chicken Salad

Prep time: 15 minutes / Cook time: 0 minutes / Serves 4

- 2 cups shredded rotisserie chicken
- 1½ tablespoons plain low-fat Greek yogurt
- ⅛ teaspoon freshly ground black pepper
- ¼ cup halved purple seedless grapes
- 8 cups chopped romaine lettuce
- 1 medium tomato, sliced
- 1 avocado, sliced

1. In a large bowl, combine the chicken, yogurt, and pepper, and mix well.
2. Stir in the grapes.
3. Divide the lettuce into four portions. Spoon one-quarter of the chicken salad onto each portion and top with a couple slices of tomato and avocado.

Per Serving:calorie: 305 / fat: 19g / protein: 24g / carbs: 11g / sugars: 4g / fiber: 6g / sodium: 79mg

Turkey Bolognese with Chickpea Pasta

Prep time: 5 minutes / Cook time: 25 minutes / Serves 4

- 1 onion, coarsely chopped
- 1 large carrot, coarsely chopped
- 2 celery stalks, coarsely chopped
- 1 tablespoon extra-virgin olive oil
- 1 pound ground turkey
- ½ cup milk
- ¾ cup red or white wine
- 1 (28-ounce) can diced tomatoes
- 10 ounces cooked chickpea pasta

1. Place the onion, carrots, and celery in a food processor and pulse until finely chopped.
2. Heat the extra-virgin olive oil in a Dutch oven or medium skillet over medium-high heat. Sauté the chopped vegetables for 3 to 5 minutes, or until softened. Add the ground turkey, breaking the poultry into smaller pieces, and cook for 5 minutes.
3. Add the milk and wine and cook until the liquid is nearly evaporated (turn up the heat to high to quicken the process).
4. Add the tomatoes and bring the sauce to a simmer. Reduce the heat to low and simmer for 10 to 15 minutes.
5. Meanwhile, cook the pasta according to the package instructions and set aside.
6. Serve the sauce with the cooked chickpea pasta.
7. Store any leftovers in an airtight container in the refrigerator for 3 to 4 days.

Per Serving:calorie: 419 / fat: 15g / protein: 31g / carbs: 34g / sugars: 8g / fiber: 11g / sodium: 150mg

Teriyaki Chicken and Broccoli

Prep time: 5 minutes / Cook time: 20 minutes / Serves 4

- For The Sauce
- ½ cup water
- 2 tablespoons low-sodium soy sauce
- 2 tablespoons honey
- 1 tablespoon rice vinegar
- ¼ teaspoon garlic powder
- Pinch ground ginger
- 1 tablespoon cornstarch
- For The Entrée
- 1 tablespoon sesame oil
- 4 (4 ounces) boneless, skinless chicken breasts, cut into bite-size cubes
- 1 (12 ounces) bag frozen broccoli
- 1 (12 ounces) bag frozen cauliflower rice

1. In a small saucepan, whisk together the water, soy sauce, honey, rice vinegar, garlic powder, and ginger. Add the cornstarch and whisk until it is fully incorporated.
2. Over medium heat, bring the teriyaki sauce to a boil. Let the sauce boil for 1 minute to thicken. Remove the sauce from the heat and set aside.

Make The Entrée 1. Heat a large skillet over medium-low heat. When hot, add the oil and the chicken. Cook for 5 to 7 minutes, until the chicken is cooked through, stirring as needed.

2. Steam the broccoli and cauliflower rice in the microwave according to the package instructions.

3. Divide the cauliflower rice into four equal portions. Put one-quarter of the broccoli and chicken over each portion and top with the teriyaki sauce.

Per Serving:calorie: 256 / fat: 7g / protein: 30g / carbs: 20g / sugars: 11g / fiber: 4g / sodium: 347mg

Wild Rice and Turkey Casserole

Prep time: 10 minutes / Cook time: 55 minutes / Serves 6

• 2 cups cut-up cooked turkey or chicken
• 2¼ cups boiling water
• ⅓ cup fat-free (skim) milk
• 4 medium green onions, sliced (¼ cup)
• 1 can (10¾ ounces) condensed 98% fat-free cream of mushroom soup
• 1 package (6 ounces) original long-grain and wild rice mix
• Additional green onions, if desired

1. Heat oven to 350°F. In ungreased 2-quart casserole, mix all ingredients, including seasoning packet from rice mix.

2. Cover; bake 45 to 50 minutes or until rice is tender. Uncover; bake 10 to 15 minutes longer or until liquid is absorbed. Sprinkle with additional green onions.

Per Serving:calories: 220 / fat: 5g / protein: 17g / carbs: 27g / sugars: 2g / fiber: 1g / sodium: 740mg

Ginger Curry Chicken Kabobs

Prep time: 5 minutes / Cook time: 5 minutes / Serves 4

• 4 teaspoons fresh lemon juice
• ½ teaspoon cayenne pepper
• ¼ teaspoon freshly ground black pepper
• 1-inch piece of fresh ginger, peeled and minced
• 1 teaspoon curry powder
• 4 teaspoons extra-virgin olive oil
• Two 8-ounce boneless, skinless chicken breasts, halved and cut into ¼-inch strips

1. In a medium bowl, combine all ingredients except the chicken. Add the chicken, and let marinate overnight in the refrigerator.

2. Thread the chicken onto metal or wooden skewers (remember to soak the wooden skewers in water before using).

3. Grill over medium heat until the chicken is no longer pink, about 15 minutes. Transfer to a platter, and serve.

Per Serving:calorie: 180 / fat: 8g / protein: 26g / carbs:

1g / sugars: 0g / fiber: 0g / sodium: 52mg

Grilled Lemon Mustard Chicken

Prep time: 5 minutes / Cook time: 15 minutes / Serves 6

• Juice of 6 medium lemons
• ½ cup mustard seeds
• 1 tablespoon minced fresh tarragon
• 2 tablespoons freshly ground black pepper
• 4 garlic cloves, minced
• 2 tablespoons extra-virgin olive oil
• Three 8-ounce boneless, skinless chicken breasts, halved

1. In a small mixing bowl, combine the lemon juice, mustard seeds, tarragon, pepper, garlic, and oil; mix well.

2. Place the chicken in a baking dish, and pour the marinade on top. Cover, and refrigerate overnight.

3. Grill the chicken over medium heat for 10–15 minutes, basting with the marinade. Serve hot.

Per Serving:calorie: 239 / fat: 11g / protein: 28g / carbs: 8g / sugars: 2g / fiber: 2g / sodium: 54mg

Rosemary Chicken with Potatoes and Green Beans

Prep time: 5 minutes / Cook time: 30 minutes / Serves 4

• ⅓ cup low-sodium chicken broth
• ¼ cup extra-virgin olive oil
• ½ teaspoon salt
• ½ teaspoon freshly ground black pepper
• ¼ teaspoon garlic powder
• ¼ teaspoon dried thyme
• 1 teaspoon dried rosemary
• 4 (4-ounce) boneless, skinless chicken breasts
• 4 small gold potatoes, cubed
• 1 pound green beans

1. Preheat the oven to 400ºF.

2. In a large bowl, whisk together the broth, oil, salt, pepper, garlic powder, thyme, and rosemary.

3. Add the chicken and potatoes to the marinade and coat well. Reserving the marinade, use a slotted spoon to remove the chicken and potatoes.

4. Arrange the chicken and potatoes on a baking sheet in a single layer and roast for 15 minutes.

5. Meanwhile, trim the green bean ends, if necessary, and put the beans in the reserved marinade.

6. Remove the baking sheet from the oven, flip the chicken breasts over, and add the green beans to the baking sheet. Pour the remaining marinade over the chicken.

7. Bake for 10 to 12 minutes until the chicken is cooked through, then broil for 2 minutes for a crisp, brown crust.

Per Serving:calorie: 426 / fat: 17g / protein: 31g / carbs:

38g / sugars: 5g / fiber: 7g / sodium: 365mg

Jerk Chicken Thighs

Prep time: 30 minutes / Cook time: 15 to 20 minutes / Serves 6

- 2 teaspoons ground coriander
- 1 teaspoon ground allspice
- 1 teaspoon cayenne pepper
- 1 teaspoon ground ginger
- 1 teaspoon salt
- 1 teaspoon dried thyme
- ½ teaspoon ground cinnamon
- ½ teaspoon ground nutmeg
- 2 pounds (907 g) boneless chicken thighs, skin on
- 2 tablespoons olive oil

1. In a small bowl, combine the coriander, allspice, cayenne, ginger, salt, thyme, cinnamon, and nutmeg. Stir until thoroughly combined.
2. Place the chicken in a baking dish and use paper towels to pat dry. Thoroughly coat both sides of the chicken with the spice mixture. Cover and refrigerate for at least 2 hours, preferably overnight.
3. Preheat the air fryer to 360°F (182°C).
4. Working in batches if necessary, arrange the chicken in a single layer in the air fryer basket and lightly coat with the olive oil. Pausing halfway through the cooking time to flip the chicken, air fry for 15 to 20 minutes, until a thermometer inserted into the thickest part registers 165°F (74°C).

Per Serving:calorie: 377 / fat: 24g / protein: 35g / carbs: 3g / sugars: 0g / fiber: 1g / sodium: 583mg

Spice-Rubbed Turkey Breast

Prep time: 5 minutes / Cook time: 45 to 55 minutes / Serves 10

- 1 tablespoon sea salt
- 1 teaspoon paprika
- 1 teaspoon onion powder
- 1 teaspoon garlic powder
- ½ teaspoon freshly ground black pepper

4 pounds (1. 8 kg) bone-in, skin-on turkey breast
- 2 tablespoons unsalted butter, melted

1. In a small bowl, combine the salt, paprika, onion powder, garlic powder, and pepper.
2. Sprinkle the seasonings all over the turkey. Brush the turkey with some of the melted butter.
3. Set the air fryer to 350°F (177°C). Place the turkey in the air fryer basket, skin-side down, and roast for 25 minutes.
4. Flip the turkey and brush it with the remaining butter. Continue cooking for another 20 to 30 minutes, until an instant-read thermometer reads 160°F (71°C).

5. Remove the turkey breast from the air fryer. Tent a piece of aluminum foil over the turkey, and allow it to rest for about 5 minutes before serving.

Per Serving:calorie: 331 / fat: 12g / protein: 49g / carbs: 2g / sugars: 0g / fiber: 1g / sodium: 2235mg

Smothered Dijon Chicken

Prep time: 10 minutes / Cook time: 30 minutes / Serves 4

- ¾ cup low-fat buttermilk
- 2 tablespoons Dijon mustard
- 3 garlic cloves, minced
- 1 tablespoon dried dill
- 1 teaspoon mustard seeds
- 2 boneless, skinless chicken breasts
- 2 large carrots, peeled and halved
- 1 medium onion, quartered

1. Preheat the oven to 375°F.
2. In a medium bowl, combine the buttermilk, mustard, garlic, dill, and mustard seeds. Mix well.
3. Add the chicken, carrots, and onion, coating them thoroughly with the buttermilk mixture. Set aside to marinate for at least 15 minutes.
4. Place the chicken, carrots, and onions on a rimmed baking sheet. Discard the remaining buttermilk mixture.
5. Transfer the baking sheet to the oven, and bake for 30 minutes, or until the vegetables are tender, and the chicken is cooked through and its juices run clear. Serve warm and enjoy.

Per Serving:calorie: 223 / fat: 5g / protein: 34g / carbs: 10g / sugars: 5g / fiber: 2g / sodium: 261mg

Chicken with Mushroom Cream Sauce

Prep time: 5 minutes / Cook time: 20 minutes / Serves 8

- 1 tablespoon extra-virgin olive oil
- Eight 3-ounce boneless, skinless chicken breast halves
- ½ cup sliced mushrooms
- 3 tablespoons flour
- ½ cup low-sodium chicken broth
- ¾ cup white wine
- 2 teaspoons lemon zest
- ½ teaspoons lemon pepper
- 1 cup plain fat-free Greek yogurt
- Parsley sprigs

1. In a large nonstick skillet, heat the oil; add the chicken and cook for 5 minutes on each side. Remove the chicken, and keep warm. Add the mushrooms to the skillet, and cook until tender.
2. In a small bowl, whisk the flour with the broth and wine. Stir the mixture into the skillet, and add the lemon zest and pepper. Cook until thickened and bubbly.
3. Return the chicken to the skillet, and cook until the chicken is no longer pink. Transfer the chicken to a platter. Stir the yogurt into the skillet and heat

thoroughly. Pour the sauce over the chicken, and garnish with parsley.

Per Serving:calorie: 166 / fat: 4g / protein: 22g / carbs: 6g / sugars: 3g / fiber: 0g / sodium: 68mg

Chicken Legs with Leeks

Prep time: 30 minutes / Cook time: 18 minutes / Serves 6

- 2 leeks, sliced
- 2 large-sized tomatoes, chopped
- 3 cloves garlic, minced
- ½ teaspoon dried oregano
- 6 chicken legs, boneless and skinless
- ½ teaspoon smoked cayenne pepper
- 2 tablespoons olive oil
- A freshly ground nutmeg

1. In a mixing dish, thoroughly combine all ingredients, minus the leeks. Place in the refrigerator and let it marinate overnight.
2. Lay the leeks onto the bottom of the air fryer basket. Top with the chicken legs.
3. Roast chicken legs at 375°F (191°C) for 18 minutes, turning halfway through. Serve with hoisin sauce.

Per Serving:calorie: 271 / fat: 12g / protein: 33g / carbs: 9g / sugars: 4g / fiber: 2g / sodium: 263mg

Pizza in a Pot

Prep time: 25 minutes / Cook time: 15 minutes / Serves 8

- 1 pound bulk lean sweet Italian turkey sausage, browned and drained
- 28 ounces can crushed tomatoes
- 15½ ounces can chili beans
- 2¼ ounces can sliced black olives, drained
- 1 medium onion, chopped
- 1 small green bell pepper, chopped
- 2 garlic cloves, minced
- ¼ cup grated Parmesan cheese
- 1 tablespoon quick-cooking tapioca
- 1 tablespoon dried basil
- 1 bay leaf

1. Set the Instant Pot to Sauté, then add the turkey sausage. Sauté until browned.
2. Add the remaining ingredients into the Instant Pot and stir.
3. Secure the lid and make sure the vent is set to sealing. Cook on Manual for 15 minutes.
4. When cook time is up, let the pressure release naturally for 5 minutes then perform a quick release. Discard bay leaf.

Per Serving:calorie: 251 / fat: 10g / protein: 18g / carbs: 23g / sugars: 8g / fiber: 3g / sodium: 936mg

Greek Chicken Stuffed Peppers

Prep time: 5 minutes / Cook time: 30 minutes / Serves 4

- 2 large red bell peppers
- 2 teaspoons extra-virgin olive oil, divided
- ½ cup uncooked brown rice or quinoa
- 4 (4-ounce) boneless, skinless chicken breasts
- ¼ teaspoon garlic powder
- ¼ teaspoon onion powder
- ⅛ teaspoon dried thyme
- ½ teaspoon dried oregano
- ½ cup crumbled feta

1. Cut the bell peppers in half and remove the seeds.
2. In a large skillet, heat 1 teaspoon of olive oil over low heat. When hot, place the bell pepper halves cut-side up in the skillet. Cover and cook for 20 minutes.
3. Cook the rice according to the package instructions.
4. Meanwhile, cut the chicken into 1-inch pieces.
5. In a medium skillet, heat the remaining 1 teaspoon of olive oil over medium-low heat. When hot, add the chicken.
6. Season the chicken with the garlic powder, onion powder, thyme, and oregano.
7. Cook for 5 minutes, stirring occasionally, until cooked through.
8. In a large bowl, combine the cooked rice and chicken. Scoop one-quarter of the chicken and rice mixture into each pepper half, cover, and cook for 10 minutes over low heat.
9. Top each pepper half with 2 tablespoons of crumbled feta.

Per Serving:calorie: 311 / fat: 11g / protein: 32g / carbs: 20g / sugars: 4g / fiber: 3g / sodium: 228mg

Creamy Garlic Chicken with Broccoli

Prep time: 5 minutes / Cook time: 15 minutes / Serves 4

- ½ cup uncooked brown rice or quinoa
- 4 (4-ounce) boneless, skinless chicken breasts
- ¼ teaspoon salt
- ¼ teaspoon freshly ground black pepper
- 1 teaspoon garlic powder, divided
- Avocado oil cooking spray
- 3 cups fresh or frozen broccoli florets
- 1 cup half-and-half

1. Cook the rice according to the package instructions.
2. Meanwhile, season both sides of the chicken breasts with the salt, pepper, and ½ teaspoon of garlic powder.
3. Heat a large skillet over medium-low heat. When hot, coat the cooking surface with cooking spray and add the chicken and broccoli in a single layer.
4. Cook for 4 minutes, then flip the chicken breasts over and cover. Cook for 5 minutes more.

5. Add the half-and-half and remaining ½ teaspoon of garlic powder to the skillet and stir. Increase the heat to high and simmer for 2 minutes.
6. Divide the rice into four equal portions. Top each portion with 1 chicken breast and one-quarter of the broccoli and cream sauce.

Per Serving:calorie: 274 / fat: 5g / protein: 31g / carbs: 27g / sugars: 3g / fiber: 1g / sodium: 271mg

One-Pan Chicken Dinner

Prep time: 5 minutes / Cook time: 35 minutes / Serves 4

- 3 tablespoons extra-virgin olive oil
- 1 tablespoon red wine vinegar or apple cider vinegar
- ¼ teaspoon garlic powder
- 3 tablespoons Italian seasoning
- 4 (4-ounce) boneless, skinless chicken breasts
- 2 cups cubed sweet potatoes
- 20 Brussels sprouts, halved lengthwise

1. Preheat the oven to 400°F.
2. In a large bowl, whisk together the oil, vinegar, garlic powder, and Italian seasoning.
3. Add the chicken, sweet potatoes, and Brussels sprouts, and coat thoroughly with the marinade.
4. Remove the ingredients from the marinade and arrange them on a baking sheet in a single layer. Roast for 15 minutes.
5. Remove the baking sheet from the oven, flip the chicken over, and bake for another 15 to 20 minutes.

Per Serving:calorie: 346 / fat: 13g / protein: 30g / carbs: 26g / sugars: 6g / fiber: 7g / sodium: 575mg

Spicy Chicken Cacciatore

Prep time: 20 minutes / Cook time: 1 hour / Serves 6

- 1 (2-pound) chicken
- ¼ cup all-purpose flour
- Sea salt
- Freshly ground black pepper
- 2 tablespoons extra-virgin olive oil
- 3 slices bacon, chopped
- 1 sweet onion, chopped
- 2 teaspoons minced garlic
- 4 ounces button mushrooms, halved
- 1 (28-ounce) can low-sodium stewed tomatoes
- ½ cup red wine
- 2 teaspoons chopped fresh oregano
- Pinch red pepper flakes

1. Cut the chicken into pieces: 2 drumsticks, 2 thighs, 2 wings, and 4 breast pieces.
2. Dredge the chicken pieces in the flour and season each piece with salt and pepper.
3. Place a large skillet over medium-high heat and add the olive oil.
4. Brown the chicken pieces on all sides, about 20

minutes in total. Transfer the chicken to a plate.
5. Add the chopped bacon to the skillet and cook until crispy, about 5 minutes. With a slotted spoon, transfer the cooked bacon to the same plate as the chicken.
6. Pour off most of the oil from the skillet, leaving just a light coating. Sauté the onion, garlic, and mushrooms in the skillet until tender, about 4 minutes.
7. Stir in the tomatoes, wine, oregano, and red pepper flakes.
8. Bring the sauce to a boil. Return the chicken and bacon, plus any accumulated juices from the plate, to the skillet.
9. Reduce the heat to low and simmer until the chicken is tender, about 30 minutes.

Per Serving:calorie: 330 / fat: 14g / protein: 35g / carbs: 14g / sugars: 7g / fiber: 4g / sodium: 196mg

Smoky Whole Chicken

Prep time: 20 minutes / Cook time: 21 minutes / Serves 6

- 2 tablespoons extra-virgin olive oil
- 1 tablespoon kosher salt
- 1½ teaspoons smoked paprika
- 1 teaspoon freshly ground black pepper
- ½ teaspoon herbes de Provence
- ¼ teaspoon cayenne pepper
- 1 (3½ pounds) whole chicken, rinsed and patted dry, giblets removed
- 1 large lemon, halved
- 6 garlic cloves, peeled and crushed with the flat side of a knife
- 1 large onion, cut into 8 wedges, divided
- 1 cup Chicken Bone Broth, low-sodium store-bought chicken broth, or water
- 2 large carrots, each cut into 4 pieces
- 2 celery stalks, each cut into 4 pieces

1. In a small bowl, combine the olive oil, salt, paprika, pepper, herbes de Provence, and cayenne.
2. Place the chicken on a cutting board and rub the olive oil mixture under the skin and all over the outside. Stuff the cavity with the lemon halves, garlic cloves, and 3 to 4 wedges of onion.
3. Pour the broth into the electric pressure cooker. Add the remaining onion wedges, carrots, and celery. Insert a wire rack or trivet on top of the vegetables.
4. Place the chicken, breast-side up, on the rack.
5. Close and lock the lid of the pressure cooker. Set the valve to sealing.
6. Cook on high pressure for 21 minutes.
7. When the cooking is complete, hit Cancel and allow the pressure to release naturally for 15 minutes, then quick release any remaining pressure.
8. Once the pin drops, unlock and remove the lid.
9. Carefully remove the chicken to a clean cutting board. Remove the skin and cut the chicken into

pieces or shred/chop the meat, and serve.

*Per Serving:*calorie: 362 / fat: 9g / protein: 60g / carbs: 8g / sugars: 3g / fiber: 2g / sodium: 611mg

Baked Chicken Dijon

Prep time: 25 minutes / Cook time: 40 minutes / Serves 6

- 3 cups uncooked bow-tie (farfalle) pasta (6 ounces)
- 2 cups frozen broccoli cuts (from 12 ounces bag)
- 2 cups cubed cooked chicken
- ⅓ cup diced roasted red bell peppers (from 7 ounces jar)
- 1 can (10¾ ounces) condensed cream of chicken or cream of mushroom soup
- ⅓ cup reduced-sodium chicken broth (from 32 ounces carton)
- 3 tablespoons Dijon mustard
- 1 tablespoon finely chopped onion
- ½ cup shredded Parmesan cheese

1. Heat oven to 375°F. Spray 2½-quart casserole with cooking spray.
2. Cook pasta as directed on package, adding broccoli for the last 2 minutes of cooking time; drain. In casserole, mix chicken and roasted peppers. In small bowl, mix soup, broth, mustard and onion; stir into chicken mixture. Stir in pasta and broccoli. Sprinkle with cheese.
3. Cover; bake about 30 minutes or until hot in center and cheese is melted.

*Per Serving:*calories: 290 / fat: 9g / protein: 24g / carbs: 29g / sugars: 2g / fiber: 3g / sodium: 770mg

Italian Chicken Thighs

Prep time: 5 minutes / Cook time: 20 minutes / Serves 2

- 4 bone-in, skin-on chicken thighs
- 2 tablespoons unsalted butter, melted
- 1 teaspoon dried parsley
- 1 teaspoon dried basil
- ½ teaspoon garlic powder
- ¼ teaspoon onion powder
- ¼ teaspoon dried oregano

1. Brush chicken thighs with butter and sprinkle remaining ingredients over thighs. Place thighs into the air fryer basket.
2. Adjust the temperature to 380ºF (193ºC) and roast for 20 minutes.
3. Halfway through the cooking time, flip the thighs.
4. When fully cooked, internal temperature will be at least 165ºF (74ºC) and skin will be crispy. Serve warm.

*Per Serving:*calorie: 446 / fat: 34g / protein: 33g / carbs: 2g / sugars: 0g / fiber: 0g / sodium: 163mg

Tangy Barbecue Strawberry-Peach Chicken

Prep time: 20 minutes / Cook time: 40 minutes / Serves 4

- For the barbecue sauce
- 1 cup frozen peaches
- 1 cup frozen strawberries
- ¼ cup tomato purée
- ½ cup white vinegar
- 1 tablespoon yellow mustard
- 1 teaspoon mustard seeds
- 1 teaspoon turmeric
- 1 teaspoon sweet paprika
- 1 teaspoon garlic powder
- ½ teaspoon cayenne pepper
- ½ teaspoon onion powder
- ½ teaspoon freshly ground black pepper
- 1 teaspoon celery seeds
- For the chicken
- 4 boneless, skinless chicken thighs

To make the barbecue sauce 1. In a stockpot, combine the peaches, strawberries, tomato purée, vinegar, mustard, mustard seeds, turmeric, paprika, garlic powder, cayenne, onion powder, black pepper, and celery seeds. Cook over low heat for 15 minutes, or until the flavors come together.
2. Remove the sauce from the heat, and let cool for 5 minutes.
3. Transfer the sauce to a blender, and purée until smooth.

To make the chicken 1. Preheat the oven to 350°F.
2. Put the chicken in a medium bowl. Coat well with ½ cup of barbecue sauce.
3. Place the chicken on a rimmed baking sheet.
4. Place the baking sheet on the middle rack of the oven, and bake for about 20 minutes (depending on the thickness of thighs), or until the juices run clear.
5. Brush the chicken with additional sauce, return to the oven, and broil on high for 3 to 5 minutes, or until a light crust forms.
6. Serve.

*Per Serving:*calorie: 389 / fat: 8g / protein: 63g / carbs: 13g / sugars: 7g / fiber: 3g / sodium: 175mg

Chicken Patties

Prep time: 15 minutes / Cook time: 12 minutes / Serves 4

- 1 pound (454 g) ground chicken thigh meat
- ½ cup shredded Mozzarella cheese
- 1 teaspoon dried parsley
- ½ teaspoon garlic powder
- ¼ teaspoon onion powder
- 1 large egg
- 2 ounces (57 g) pork rinds, finely ground

1. In a large bowl, mix ground chicken, Mozzarella, parsley, garlic powder, and onion powder. Form into four patties.
2. Place patties in the freezer for 15 to 20 minutes until they begin to firm up.
3. Whisk egg in a medium bowl. Place the ground pork rinds into a large bowl.
4. Dip each chicken patty into the egg and then press into pork rinds to fully coat. Place patties into the air fryer basket.
5. Adjust the temperature to 360ºF (182ºC) and air fry for 12 minutes.
6. Patties will be firm and cooked to an internal temperature of 165ºF (74ºC) when done. Serve immediately.

*Per Serving:*calorie: 394 / fat: 26g / protein: 35g / carbs: 2g / sugars: 0g / fiber: 0g / sodium: 563mg

Sesame-Ginger Chicken Soba

Prep time: 10 minutes / Cook time: 15 minutes / Serves 6

- 8 ounces soba noodles
- 2 boneless, skinless chicken breasts, halved lengthwise
- ¼ cup tahini
- 2 tablespoons rice vinegar
- 1 tablespoon reduced-sodium gluten-free soy sauce or tamari
- 1 teaspoon toasted sesame oil
- 1 (1-inch) piece fresh ginger, finely grated
- ⅓ cup water
- 1 large cucumber, seeded and diced
- 1 scallions bunch, green parts only, cut into 1-inch segments
- 1 tablespoon sesame seeds

1. Preheat the broiler to high.
2. Bring a large pot of water to a boil. Add the noodles and cook until tender, according to the package directions. Drain and rinse the noodles in cool water.
3. On a baking sheet, arrange the chicken in a single layer. Broil for 5 to 7 minutes on each side, depending on the thickness, until the chicken is cooked through and its juices run clear. Use two forks to shred the chicken.
4. In a small bowl, combine the tahini, rice vinegar, soy sauce, sesame oil, ginger, and water. Whisk to combine.
5. In a large bowl, toss the shredded chicken, noodles, cucumber, and scallions. Pour the tahini sauce over the noodles and toss to combine. Served sprinkled with the sesame seeds.

*Per Serving:*calories: 251 / fat: 8g / protein: 16g / carbs: 35g / sugars: 2g / fiber: 2g / sodium: 482mg

Asian Mushroom-Chicken Soup

Prep time: 30 minutes / Cook time: 15 minutes / Serves 6

- 1½ cups water
- 1 package (1 ounce) dried portabella or shiitake mushrooms
- 1 tablespoon canola oil
- ¼ cup thinly sliced green onions (4 medium)
- 2 tablespoons gingerroot, peeled, minced
- 3 cloves garlic, minced
- 1 jalapeño chile, seeded, minced
- 1 cup fresh snow pea pods, sliced diagonally
- 3 cups reduced-sodium chicken broth
- 1 can (8 ounces) sliced bamboo shoots, drained
- 2 tablespoons low-sodium soy sauce
- ½ teaspoon sriracha sauce
- 1 cup shredded cooked chicken breast
- 1 cup cooked brown rice
- 4 teaspoons lime juice
- ½ cup thinly sliced fresh basil leaves

1. In medium microwavable bowl, heat water uncovered on High 30 seconds or until hot. Add mushrooms; let stand 5 minutes or until tender. Drain mushrooms (reserve liquid). Slice any mushrooms that are large. Set aside.
2. In 4-quart saucepan, heat oil over medium heat. Add 2 tablespoons of the green onions, the gingerroot, garlic and chile to oil. Cook about 3 minutes, stirring occasionally, until vegetables are tender. Add snow pea pods; cook 2 minutes, stirring occasionally. Stir in mushrooms, reserved mushroom liquid and the remaining ingredients, except lime juice and basil. Heat to boiling; reduce heat. Cover and simmer 10 minutes or until hot. Stir in lime juice.
3. Divide soup evenly among 6 bowls. Top servings with basil and remaining green onions.

*Per Serving:*calories: 150 / fat: 4g / protein: 11g / carbs: 16g / sugars: 3g / fiber: 3g / sodium: 490mg

Grain-Free Parmesan Chicken

Prep time: 5 minutes / Cook time: 20 minutes / Serves 4

- 1½ cups (144 g) almond flour
- ½ cup (50 g) grated Parmesan cheese
- 1 tablespoon (3 g) Italian seasoning
- 1 teaspoon garlic powder
- ½ teaspoon black pepper
- 2 large eggs
- 4 (6 ounces [170 g], ½-inch [13 mm]-thick) boneless, skinless chicken breasts
- ½ cup (120 ml) no-added-sugar marinara sauce
- ½ cup (56 g) shredded mozzarella cheese
- 2 tablespoons (8 g) minced fresh herbs of choice (optional)

1. Preheat the oven to 375°F (191°C). Line a large, rimmed baking sheet with parchment paper.
2. In a shallow dish, mix together the almond flour, Parmesan cheese, Italian seasoning, garlic powder, and black pepper. In another shallow dish, whisk the eggs. Dip a chicken breast into the egg wash, then gently shake off any extra egg. Dip the chicken breast into the almond flour mixture, coating it well. Place the chicken breast on the prepared baking sheet. Repeat this process with the remaining chicken breasts.
3. Bake the chicken for 15 to 20 minutes, or until the meat is no longer pink in the center.
4. Remove the chicken from the oven and flip each breast. Top each breast with 2 tablespoons (30 ml) of marinara sauce and 2 tablespoons (14 g) of mozzarella cheese.
5. Increase the oven temperature to broil and place the chicken back in the oven. Broil it until the cheese is melted and just starting to brown. Carefully remove the chicken from the oven, top it with the herbs (if using), and let it rest for about 10 minutes before serving.

Per Serving:calorie: 572 / fat: 32g / protein: 60g / carbs: 13g / sugars: 4g / fiber:5g / sodium: 560mg

Peanut Chicken Satay

Prep time: 20 minutes / Cook time: 10 minutes / Serves 8

- For The Peanut Sauce
- 1 cup natural peanut butter
- 2 tablespoons low-sodium tamari or gluten-free soy sauce
- 1 teaspoon red chili paste
- 1 tablespoon honey
- Juice of 2 limes
- ½ cup hot water
- For The Chicken
- 2 pounds boneless, skinless chicken thighs, trimmed of fat and cut into 1-inch pieces
- ½ cup plain nonfat Greek yogurt
- 2 garlic cloves, minced
- 1 teaspoon minced fresh ginger
- ½ onion, coarsely chopped
- 1½ teaspoons ground coriander
- 2 teaspoons ground cumin
- ½ teaspoon salt
- 1 teaspoon extra-virgin olive oil
- Lettuce leaves, for serving

Make The Peanut Sauce: 1. In a medium mixing bowl, combine the peanut butter, tamari, chili paste, honey, lime juice, and hot water. Mix until smooth. Set aside.

Make The Chicken: 1. In a large mixing bowl, combine the chicken, yogurt, garlic, ginger, onion,

coriander, cumin, and salt, and mix well.
2. Cover and marinate in the refrigerator for at least 2 hours.
3. Thread the chicken pieces onto bamboo skewers.
4. In a grill pan or large skillet, heat the oil. Cook the skewers for 3 to 5 minutes on each side until the pieces are cooked through.
5. Remove the chicken from the skewers and place a few pieces on each lettuce leaf. Drizzle with the peanut sauce and serve.

Per Serving:calories: 386/ fat: 26g / protein: 16g / carbs: 14g / sugars: 6g / fiber: 2g / sodium: 442mg

Taco Stuffed Sweet Potatoes

Prep time: 5 minutes / Cook time: 15 minutes / Serves 4

- 4 medium sweet potatoes
- 2 tablespoons extra-virgin olive oil
- 1 pound 93% lean ground turkey
- 2 teaspoons ground cumin
- 1 teaspoon chili powder
- ½ teaspoon salt
- ½ teaspoon freshly ground black pepper

1. Pierce the potatoes with a fork, and microwave them on the potato setting, or for 10 minutes on high power.
2. Meanwhile, heat a medium skillet over medium heat. When hot, put the oil, turkey, cumin, chili powder, salt, and pepper into the skillet, stirring and breaking apart the meat, as needed.
3. Remove the potatoes from the microwave and halve them lengthwise. Depress the centers with a spoon, and fill each half with an equal amount of cooked turkey.

Per Serving:calorie: 348 / fat: 17g / protein: 24g / carbs: 27g / sugars: 6g / fiber: 4g / sodium: 462mg

Chicken Nuggets

Prep time: 10 minutes / Cook time: 15 minutes / Serves 4

- 1 pound (454 g) ground chicken thighs
- ½ cup shredded Mozzarella cheese
- 1 large egg, whisked
- ½ teaspoon salt
- ¼ teaspoon dried oregano
- ¼ teaspoon garlic powder

1. In a large bowl, combine all ingredients. Form mixture into twenty nugget shapes, about 2 tablespoons each.
2. Place nuggets into ungreased air fryer basket, working in batches if needed. Adjust the temperature to 375°F (191°C) and air fry for 15 minutes, turning nuggets halfway through cooking. Let cool 5 minutes before serving.

Per Serving:calorie: 315 / fat: 19g / protein: 30g / carbs: 2g / sugars: 0g / fiber: 0g / sodium: 495mg

Chapter 4 Beef, Pork, and Lamb

Garlic Beef Stroganoff

Prep time: 20 minutes / Cook time: 25 minutes / Serves 6

- 2 tablespoons canola oil
- 1½ pounds boneless round steak, cut into thin strips, trimmed of fat
- 2 teaspoons sodium-free beef bouillon powder
- 1 cup mushroom juice, with water added to make a full cup
- 2 (4½ ounces) jars sliced mushrooms, drained with juice reserved
- 10¾ ounces can 98% fat-free, lower-sodium cream of mushroom soup
- 1 large onion, chopped
- 3 garlic cloves, minced
- 1 tablespoon Worcestershire sauce
- 6 ounces fat-free cream cheese, cubed and softened

1. Press the Sauté button and put the oil into the Instant Pot inner pot.
2. Once the oil is heated, sauté the beef until it is lightly browned, about 2 minutes on each side. Set the beef aside for a moment. Press Cancel and wipe out the Instant Pot with some paper towel.
3. Press Sauté again and dissolve the bouillon in the mushroom juice and water in inner pot of the Instant Pot. Once dissolved, press Cancel.
4. Add the mushrooms, soup, onion, garlic, and Worcestershire sauce and stir. Add the beef back to the pot.
5. Secure the lid and make sure the vent is set to sealing. Press Manual and set for 15 minutes.
6. When cook time is up, let the pressure release naturally for 15 minutes, then perform a quick release.
7. Press Cancel and remove the lid. Press Sauté. Stir in cream cheese until smooth.
8. Serve over noodles.

Per Serving:*calories: 202 / fat: 8g / protein: 21g / carbs: 10g / sugars: 4g / fiber: 2g / sodium: 474mg*

Open-Faced Pulled Pork

Prep time: 15 minutes / Cook time: 1 hour 35minutes / Serves 2

- 2 tablespoons hoisin sauce
- 2 tablespoons tomato paste
- 2 tablespoons rice vinegar
- 1 tablespoon minced fresh ginger
- 2 teaspoons minced garlic
- 1 teaspoon chile-garlic sauce
- ¾ pound pork shoulder, trimmed of any visible fat, cut into 2-inch-square cubes
- 4 large romaine lettuce leaves

1. Preheat the oven to 300°F.
2. In a medium ovenproof pot with a tight-fitting lid, stir together the hoisin sauce, tomato paste, rice vinegar, ginger, garlic, and chile-garlic sauce.
3. Add the pork. Toss to coat.
4. Place the pot over medium heat. Bring to a simmer. Cover and carefully transfer the ovenproof pot to the preheated oven. Cook for 90 minutes.
5. Check the meat for doneness by inserting a fork into one of the chunks. If it goes in easily and the pork falls apart, the meat is done. If not, cook for another 30 minutes or so, until the meat passes the fork test.
6. Using a coarse strainer, strain the cooked pork into a fat separator. Shred the meat. Set aside. If you don't have a fat separator, remove the meat from the sauce and set aside. Let the sauce cool until any fat has risen to the top. With a spoon, remove as much fat as possible or use paper towels to blot it off.
7. In a small saucepan set over high heat, pour the defatted sauce. Bring to a boil, stirring frequently to prevent scorching. Cook for 2 to 3 minutes, or until thickened.
8. Add the shredded meat. Toss to coat with the sauce. Cook for 1 minute to reheat the meat.
9. Spoon equal amounts of pork into the romaine lettuce leaves and enjoy!

Per Serving:*calorie: 289 / fat: 11g / protein: 33g / carbs: 13g / sugars: 7g / fiber: 1g / sodium: 391mg*

Bone-in Pork Chops

Prep time: 5 minutes / Cook time: 10 to 12 minutes / Serves 2

- 1 pound (454 g) bone-in pork chops
- 1 tablespoon avocado oil
- 1 teaspoon smoked paprika
- ½ teaspoon onion powder
- ¼ teaspoon cayenne pepper
- Sea salt and freshly ground black pepper, to taste

1. Brush the pork chops with the avocado oil. In a small dish, mix together the smoked paprika, onion powder, cayenne pepper, and salt and black pepper to taste. Sprinkle the seasonings over both sides of the pork chops.
2. Set the air fryer to 400°F (204°C). Place the chops in the air fryer basket in a single layer, working in batches if necessary. Air fry for 10 to 12 minutes, until an instant-read thermometer reads 145°F (63°C) at the chops' thickest point.
3. Remove the chops from the air fryer and allow them to rest for 5 minutes before serving.

Per Serving:*calorie: 429 / fat: 29g / protein: 39g / carbs: 1g / sugars: 0g / fiber: 0g / sodium: 82mg*

Gingered-Pork Stir-Fry

Prep time: 10 minutes / Cook time: 20 minutes / Serves 2

- 2 tablespoons extra-virgin olive oil
- 2 garlic cloves, minced
- 1 (½-inch) piece fresh ginger, peeled, thinly sliced
- ¼ pound lean pork, thinly sliced
- 2 teaspoons low-sodium soy sauce
- 1 teaspoon granulated stevia
- 1 teaspoon sesame oil • 1 cup snow peas
- 1 medium red bell pepper, sliced
- 6 whole fresh mushrooms, sliced
- 2 scallions, chopped
- 1 tablespoon Chinese rice wine
- 2 tablespoons chopped cashews, divided

1. In a large skillet or wok set over medium-high heat, heat the olive oil.
2. Add the garlic and ginger. Sauté for 1 to 2 minutes, or until fragrant.
3. Add the pork, soy sauce, and stevia. Cook for 10 minutes, stirring occasionally.
4. Stir in the sesame oil, snow peas, bell pepper, mushrooms, scallions, and rice wine. Reduce the heat to low. Simmer for 4 to 8 minutes, or until the pork is tender.
5. Divide between 2 serving plates, sprinkle each serving with 1 tablespoon of cashews and enjoy!

Per Serving:*calorie: 365 / fat: 23g / protein: 21g / carbs: 22g / sugars: 8g / fiber: 6g / sodium: 203mg*

Salisbury Steaks with Seared Cauliflower

Prep time: 5 minutes / Cook time: 30 minutes / Serves 4

- Salisbury Steaks
- 1 pound 95 percent lean ground beef
- ⅓ cup almond flour • 1 large egg
- ½ teaspoon fine sea salt
- ¼ teaspoon freshly ground black pepper
- 2 tablespoons cold-pressed avocado oil
- 1 small yellow onion, sliced
- 1 garlic clove, chopped
- 8 ounces cremini or button mushrooms, sliced
- ½ teaspoon fine sea salt
- 2 tablespoons tomato paste
- 1½ teaspoons yellow mustard
- 1 cup low-sodium roasted beef bone broth
- Seared Cauliflower • 1 tablespoon olive oil
- 1 head cauliflower, cut into bite-size florets
- 2 tablespoons chopped fresh flat-leaf parsley
- ¼ teaspoon fine sea salt • 2 teaspoons cornstarch
- 2 teaspoons water

1. To make the steaks: In a bowl, combine the beef, almond flour, egg, salt, and pepper and mix with your hands until all of the ingredients are evenly distributed. Divide the mixture into four equal portions, then shape each portion into an oval patty about ½ inch thick.
2. Select the Sauté setting on the Instant Pot and heat the oil for 2 minutes. Swirl the oil to coat the bottom of the pot, then add the patties and sear for 3 minutes, until browned on one side. Using a thin, flexible spatula, flip the patties and sear the second side for 2 to 3 minutes, until browned. Transfer the patties to a plate.
3. Add the onion, garlic, mushrooms, and salt to the pot and sauté for 4 minutes, until the onion is translucent and the mushrooms have begun to give up their liquid. Add the tomato paste, mustard, and broth and stir with a wooden spoon, using it to nudge any browned bits from the bottom of the pot. Return the patties to the pot in a single layer and spoon a bit of the sauce over each one.
4. Secure the lid and set the Pressure Release to Sealing. Press the Cancel button to reset the cooking program, then select the Pressure Cook or Manual setting and set the cooking time for 10 minutes at high pressure. (The pot will take about 5 minutes to come up to pressure before the cooking program begins.)
5. When the cooking program ends, let the pressure release naturally for at least 10 minutes, then move the Pressure Release to Venting to release any remaining steam.
6. To make the cauliflower: While the pressure is releasing, in a large skillet over medium heat, warm the oil. Add the cauliflower and stir or toss to coat with the oil, then cook, stirring every minute or two, until lightly browned, about 8 minutes. Turn off the heat, sprinkle in the parsley and salt, and stir to combine. Leave in the skillet, uncovered, to keep warm.
7. Open the pot and, using a slotted spatula, transfer the patties to a serving plate. In a small bowl, stir together the cornstarch and water. Press the Cancel button to reset the cooking program, then select the Sauté setting. When the sauce comes to a simmer, stir in the cornstarch mixture and let the sauce boil for about 1 minute, until thickened. Press the Cancel button to turn off the Instant Pot.
8. Spoon the sauce over the patties. Serve right away, with the cauliflower.

Per Serving:*calorie: 362 / fat: 21g / protein: 33g / carbs: 21g / sugars: 4g / fiber: 6g / sodium: 846mg*

Smoky Pork Tenderloin

Prep time: 5 minutes / Cook time: 19 to 22 minutes / Serves 6

- 1½ pounds (680 g) pork tenderloin

- 1 tablespoon avocado oil• 1 teaspoon chili powder
- 1 teaspoon smoked paprika
- 1 teaspoon garlic powder • 1 teaspoon sea salt
- 1 teaspoon freshly ground black pepper

1. Pierce the tenderloin all over with a fork and rub the oil all over the meat.
2. In a small dish, stir together the chili powder, smoked paprika, garlic powder, salt, and pepper.
3. Rub the spice mixture all over the tenderloin.
4. Set the air fryer to 400ºF (204ºC). Place the pork in the air fryer basket and air fry for 10 minutes. Flip the tenderloin and cook for 9 to 12 minutes more, until an instant-read thermometer reads at least 145ºF (63ºC).
5. Allow the tenderloin to rest for 5 minutes, then slice and serve.

Per Serving:calorie: 217 / fat: 8g / protein: 34g / carbs: 1g / sugars: 0g / fiber: 0g / sodium: 414mg

Creole Steak

Prep time: 5 minutes / Cook time: 1 hour 40 minutes / Serves 4

- 2 teaspoons extra-virgin olive oil
- ¼ cup chopped onion
- ¼ cup chopped green bell pepper
- 1 cup canned crushed tomatoes
- ½ teaspoon chili powder• ¼ teaspoon celery seed
- 4 cloves garlic, finely chopped
- ¼ teaspoon salt   • 1 teaspoon cumin
- 1 pound lean boneless round steak

1. In a large skillet over medium heat, heat the oil. Add the onions and green pepper, and sauté until the onions are translucent (about 5 minutes).
2. Add the tomatoes, chili powder, celery seed, garlic, salt, and cumin; cover and let simmer over low heat for 20–25 minutes. This allows the flavors to blend.
3. Preheat the oven to 350 degrees. Trim all visible fat off the steak.
4. In a nonstick pan or a pan that has been sprayed with nonstick cooking spray, lightly brown the steak on each side. Transfer the steak to a 13-x-9-x-2-inch baking dish; pour the sauce over the steak, and cover.
5. Bake for 1¼ hours or until the steak is tender. Remove from the oven; slice the steak, and arrange on a serving platter. Spoon the sauce over the steak, and serve.

Per Serving:calorie: 213 / fat: 10g / protein: 25g / carbs: 5g / sugars: 2g / fiber: 2g / sodium: 235mg

Open-Faced Pub-Style Bison Burgers

Prep time: 10 minutes / Cook time: 15 minutes / Serves 4

- 2 tablespoons extra-virgin olive oil

- 1 onion, thinly sliced   • 1 pound ground bison
- 1 teaspoon sea salt, divided
- 1 cup blue cheese crumbles
- 4 slices sourdough bread
- 1 garlic clove, halved   • Pub Sauce

1. In a large skillet over medium-high heat, heat the olive oil until it shimmers. Add the onion. Cook, stirring, until it begins to brown, about 5 minutes.
2. Set the onion aside, and wipe out the skillet with a paper towel and return it to the stove at medium-high heat. Season the bison with the salt and form it into 4 patties. Brown the patties in the hot skillet until they reach an internal temperature of 140°F, about 5 minutes per side.
3. Sprinkle the blue cheese over the tops of the burgers and remove the skillet from the heat. Cover the skillet and allow the cheese to melt.
4. Meanwhile, toast the bread and then rub the garlic halves over the pieces of toast to flavor them.
5. To assemble, put a piece of toast on a plate. Top with onion slices, place a burger patty on top, and then spoon the sauce over the patty.

Per Serving:calorie: 433 / fat: 25g / protein: 33g / carbs: 18g / sugars: 2g / fiber: 1g / sodium: 563mg

Pork Tacos

Prep time: 30 minutes / Cook time: 10 minutes / Serves 2

- 8 ounces boneless skinless pork tenderloin, thinly sliced, ¼-inch thick, across the grain
- Pinch salt
- ⅓ cup ancho chile sauce
- 2 tablespoons chipotle purée (see Recipe Tip)
- ¼ cup freshly squeezed lime juice
- 2 (6-inch) soft low-carb corn tortillas, such as La Tortilla
- 4 tablespoons diced tomatoes, divided
- 1 cup shredded lettuce, divided
- ½ avocado, sliced   • 4 tablespoons salsa, divided

1. Sprinkle the pork slices with salt. Set aside.
2. In a small bowl, stir together the ancho chile sauce, chipotle purée, and lime juice. Reserve 3 tablespoons of the marinade. Set aside.
3. In a large sealable plastic bag, add the pork. Pour the remaining marinade over it. Seal the bag, removing as much air as possible. Marinate the meat for 20 minutes to 1 hour at room temperature, or refrigerate for several hours. Turn the meat twice while it marinates.
4. Place a small nonstick skillet over medium heat. Have a large piece of aluminum foil nearby.
5. Working with one tortilla at a time, heat both sides in the skillet until they puff slightly. As they are done, stack the tortillas on the foil. When they are all heated, wrap the tortillas in the foil.

6. Preheat the broiler.

7. Adjust the rack so it is 4 inches from the heating element.

8. Remove the pork slices from the marinade. Discard the marinade. Place the pork on a rack set over a sheet pan.

9. Place the pan in the oven. Broil for 3 to 4 minutes, or until the edges of the pork begin to brown. Remove from the oven. Turn and brush the pork with the reserved marinade. Broil the second side for 3 minutes, or until the pork is just barely pink inside.

10. Place the foil packet with the tortillas in the oven to warm while the pork finishes cooking.

11. To serve, pile each tortilla with a few slices of pork. Top each with about 2 tablespoons of diced tomato, ½ cup of shredded lettuce, half of the avocado slices, and about 2 tablespoons of salsa.

Per Serving:calorie: 328 / fat: 13g / protein: 30g / carbs: 25g / sugars: 5g / fiber: 7g / sodium: 563mg

Coffee-and-Herb-Marinated Steak

Prep time: 10 minutes / Cook time: 10 minutes / Serves 4

- ¼ cup whole coffee beans
- 2 teaspoons minced garlic
- 2 teaspoons chopped fresh rosemary
- 2 teaspoons chopped fresh thyme
- 1 teaspoon freshly ground black pepper
- 2 tablespoons apple cider vinegar
- 2 tablespoons extra-virgin olive oil
- 1 pound flank steak, trimmed of visible fat

1. Place the coffee beans, garlic, rosemary, thyme, and black pepper in a coffee grinder or food processor and pulse until coarsely ground.

2. Transfer the coffee mixture to a resealable plastic bag and add the vinegar and oil. Shake to combine.

3. Add the flank steak and squeeze the excess air out of the bag. Seal it. Marinate the steak in the refrigerator for at least 2 hours, occasionally turning the bag over.

4. Preheat the broiler. Line a baking sheet with aluminum foil.

5. Take the steak out of the bowl and discard the marinade.

6. Place the steak on the baking sheet and broil until it is done to your liking, about 5 minutes per side for medium.

7. Let the steak rest for 10 minutes before slicing it thinly on a bias.

8. Serve with a mixed green salad or your favorite side dish.

Per Serving:calorie: 191 / fat: 9g / protein: 25g / carbs: 1g / sugars: 0g / fiber: 0g / sodium: 127mg

Pork Chop Diane

Prep time: 10 minutes / Cook time: 20 minutes / Serves 4

- ¼ cup low-sodium chicken broth
- 1 tablespoon freshly squeezed lemon juice
- 2 teaspoons Worcestershire sauce
- 2 teaspoons Dijon mustard
- 4 (5-ounce) boneless pork top loin chops, about 1 inch thick
- Sea salt   • Freshly ground black pepper
- 1 teaspoon extra-virgin olive oil
- 1 teaspoon lemon zest • 1 teaspoon butter
- 2 teaspoons chopped fresh chives

1. In a small bowl, stir together the chicken broth, lemon juice, Worcestershire sauce, and Dijon mustard and set it aside.

2. Season the pork chops lightly with salt and pepper.

3. Place a large skillet over medium-high heat and add the olive oil.

4. Cook the pork chops, turning once, until they are no longer pink, about 8 minutes per side.

5. Transfer the chops to a plate and set it aside.

6. Pour the broth mixture into the skillet and cook until warmed through and thickened, about 2 minutes.

7. Whisk in the lemon zest, butter, and chives.

8. Serve the chops with a generous spoonful of sauce.

Per Serving:calorie: 203 / fat: 7g / protein: 32g / carbs: 1g / sugars: 0g / fiber: 0g / sodium: 130mg

Goat Cheese-Stuffed Flank Steak

Prep time: 10 minutes / Cook time: 14 minutes / Serves 6

- 1 pound (454 g) flank steak
- 1 tablespoon avocado oil • ½ teaspoon sea salt
- ½ teaspoon garlic powder
- ¼ teaspoon freshly ground black pepper
- 2 ounces (57 g) goat cheese, crumbled
- 1 cup baby spinach, chopped

1. Place the steak in a large zip-top bag or between two pieces of plastic wrap. Using a meat mallet or heavy-bottomed skillet, pound the steak to an even ¼-inch thickness.

2. Brush both sides of the steak with the avocado oil.

3. Mix the salt, garlic powder, and pepper in a small dish. Sprinkle this mixture over both sides of the steak.

4. Sprinkle the goat cheese over top, and top that with the spinach.

5. Starting at one of the long sides, roll the steak up tightly. Tie the rolled steak with kitchen string at 3-inch intervals.

6. Set the air fryer to 400°F (204°C). Place the steak roll-up in the air fryer basket. Air fry for 7 minutes. Flip the steak and cook for an additional 7 minutes, until an instant-read thermometer reads 120°F (49°C) for medium-rare (adjust the cooking time for your desired doneness).

Per Serving:calorie: 210 / fat: 11g / protein: 22g / carbs: 2g / sugars: 0g / fiber: 1g / sodium: 330mg

Greek Stuffed Tenderloin

Prep time: 10 minutes / Cook time: 10 minutes / Serves 4

- 1½ pounds (680 g) venison or beef tenderloin, pounded to ¼ inch thick
- 3 teaspoons fine sea salt
- 1 teaspoon ground black pepper
- 2 ounces (57 g) creamy goat cheese
- ½ cup crumbled feta cheese (about 2 ounces / 57 g)
- ¼ cup finely chopped onions
- 2 cloves garlic, minced
- For Garnish/Serving (Optional):
- Prepared yellow mustard
- Halved cherry tomatoes • Extra-virgin olive oil
- Sprigs of fresh rosemary   • Lavender flowers

1. Spray the air fryer basket with avocado oil. Preheat the air fryer to 400°F (204°C).
2. Season the tenderloin on all sides with the salt and pepper.
3. In a medium-sized mixing bowl, combine the goat cheese, feta, onions, and garlic. Place the mixture in the center of the tenderloin. Starting at the end closest to you, tightly roll the tenderloin like a jelly roll. Tie the rolled tenderloin tightly with kitchen twine.
4. Place the meat in the air fryer basket and air fry for 5 minutes. Flip the meat over and cook for another 5 minutes, or until the internal temperature reaches 135°F (57°C) for medium-rare.
5. To serve, smear a line of prepared yellow mustard on a platter, then place the meat next to it and add halved cherry tomatoes on the side, if desired. Drizzle with olive oil and garnish with rosemary sprigs and lavender flowers, if desired.
6. Best served fresh. Store leftovers in an airtight container in the fridge for 3 days. Reheat in a preheated 350°F (177°C) air fryer for 4 minutes, or until heated through.

Per Serving:calories: 345 / fat: 17g / protein: 43g / carbs: 2g / sugars: 2g / fiber: 0g / sodium: 676mg

Steak with Bell Pepper

Prep time: 30 minutes / Cook time: 20 to 23 minutes / Serves 6

- ¼ cup avocado oil
- ¼ cup freshly squeezed lime juice
- 2 teaspoons minced garlic
- 1 tablespoon chili powder
- ½ teaspoon ground cumin
- Sea salt and freshly ground black pepper, to taste
- 1 pound (454 g) top sirloin steak or flank steak, thinly sliced against the grain
- 1 red bell pepper, cored, seeded, and cut into ½-inch slices
- 1 green bell pepper, cored, seeded, and cut into ½-inch slices   • 1 large onion, sliced

1. In a small bowl or blender, combine the avocado oil, lime juice, garlic, chili powder, cumin, and salt and pepper to taste.
2. Place the sliced steak in a zip-top bag or shallow dish. Place the bell peppers and onion in a separate zip-top bag or dish. Pour half the marinade over the steak and the other half over the vegetables. Seal both bags and let the steak and vegetables marinate in the refrigerator for at least 1 hour or up to 4 hours.
3. Line the air fryer basket with an air fryer liner or aluminum foil. Remove the vegetables from their bag or dish and shake off any excess marinade. Set the air fryer to 400°F (204°C). Place the vegetables in the air fryer basket and cook for 13 minutes.
4. Remove the steak from its bag or dish and shake off any excess marinade. Place the steak on top of the vegetables in the air fryer, and cook for 7 to 10 minutes or until an instant-read thermometer reads 120°F (49°C) for medium-rare (or cook to your desired doneness).
5. Serve with desired fixings, such as keto tortillas, lettuce, sour cream, avocado slices, shredded Cheddar cheese, and cilantro.

Per Serving:calorie: 330 / fat: 24g / protein: 20g / carbs: 12g / sugars: 4g / fiber: 3g / sodium: 160mg

Pork Carnitas

Prep time: 10 minutes / Cook time: 20 minutes / Serves 8

- 1 teaspoon kosher salt
- 2 teaspoons chili powder
- 2 teaspoons dried oregano
- ½ teaspoon freshly ground black pepper
- 1 (2½-pound) pork sirloin roast or boneless pork butt, cut into 1½-inch cubes
- 2 tablespoons avocado oil, divided
- 3 garlic cloves, minced
- Juice and zest of 1 large orange
- Juice and zest of 1 medium lime
- 6-inch gluten-free corn tortillas, warmed, for serving (optional)
- Chopped avocado, for serving (optional)
- Roasted Tomatillo Salsa or salsa verde, for serving (optional)
- Shredded cheddar cheese, for serving (optional)

1. In a large bowl or gallon-size zip-top bag, combine the salt, chili powder, oregano, and pepper. Add the pork cubes and toss to coat.
2. Set the electric pressure cooker to the Sauté/More setting. When the pot is hot, pour in 1 tablespoon of avocado oil.
3. Add half of the pork to the pot and sear until the pork is browned on all sides, about 5 minutes. Transfer the pork to a plate, add the remaining 1

tablespoon of avocado oil to the pot, and sear the remaining pork. Hit Cancel.

4. Return all of the pork to the pot and add the garlic, orange zest and juice, and lime zest and juice to the pot.
5. Close and lock the lid of the pressure cooker. Set the valve to sealing.
6. Cook on high pressure for 20 minutes.
7. When the cooking is complete, hit Cancel. Allow the pressure to release naturally for 15 minutes then quick release any remaining pressure.
8. Once the pin drops, unlock and remove the lid.
9. Using two forks, shred the meat right in the pot.
10. (Optional) For more authentic carnitas, spread the shredded meat on a broiler-safe sheet pan. Preheat the broiler with the rack 6 inches from the heating element. Broil the pork for about 5 minutes or until it begins to crisp. (Watch carefully so you don't let the pork burn.) 11. Place the pork in a serving bowl. Top with some of the juices from the pot. Serve with tortillas, avocado, salsa, and Cheddar cheese (if using).

Per Serving:calorie: 218 / fat: 7g / protein: 33g / carbs: 4g / sugars: 2g / fiber: 1g / sodium: 400mg

Bavarian Beef

Prep time: 35 minutes / Cook time: 1 hour 15 minutes / Serves 8

- 1 tablespoon canola oil
- 3-pound boneless beef chuck roast, trimmed of fat
- 3 cups sliced carrots   • 3 cups sliced onions
- 2 large kosher dill pickles, chopped
- 1 cup sliced celery
- ½ cup dry red wine or beef broth
- ⅓ cup German-style mustard
- 2 teaspoons coarsely ground black pepper
- 2 bay leaves   • ¼ teaspoon ground cloves
- 1 cup water   • ⅓ cup flour

1. Press Sauté on the Instant Pot and add in the oil. Brown roast on both sides for about 5 minutes. Press Cancel.
2. Add all of the remaining ingredients, except for the flour, to the Instant Pot.
3. Secure the lid and make sure the vent is set to sealing. Press Manual and set the time to 1 hour and 15 minutes. Let the pressure release naturally.
4. Remove meat and vegetables to large platter. Cover to keep warm.
5. Remove 1 cup of the liquid from the Instant Pot and mix with the flour. Press Sauté on the Instant Pot and add the flour/broth mixture back in, whisking. Cook until the broth is smooth and thickened.
6. Serve over noodles or spaetzle.

Per Serving:calories: 251 / fat: 8g / protein: 26g / carbs: 17g / sugars: 7g / fiber: 4g / sodium: 525mg

Peppered Beef with Greens and Beans

Prep time: 10 minutes / Cook time: 20 minutes / Serves 2

- 1 (½-pound, ½-inch-thick) boneless beef sirloin, halved
- 2 teaspoons coarsely ground black pepper, divided
- ¼ cup tomato sauce
- 2 tablespoons red wine vinegar
- 1 teaspoon dried basil
- 3 cups (1 bunch) chopped kale
- 1 cup chopped green beans
- ¾ cup chopped red bell pepper, or yellow bell pepper
- ¼ cup chopped onion

1. Rub each side of the steak halves with ½ teaspoon of coarsely ground pepper.
2. Heat a 10-inch nonstick skillet over medium heat. Add the beef. Cook for 8 to 12 minutes, turning once halfway through.
3. Add the tomato sauce, red wine vinegar, and basil. Stir to combine.
4. Add the kale, green beans, bell pepper, and onion. Stir to mix with the sauce. Reduce the heat to medium-low. Cook for about 5 minutes, uncovered, or until the vegetables are tender and beef is cooked medium doneness (160°F).
5. Serve immediately and enjoy!

Per Serving:calorie: 277 / fat: 13g / protein: 27g / carbs: 13g / sugars: 6g / fiber: 5g / sodium: 80mg

Pork Meatballs

Prep time: 10 minutes / Cook time: 12 minutes / Makes 18 meatballs

- 1 pound (454 g) ground pork
- 1 large egg, whisked
- ½ teaspoon garlic powder
- ½ teaspoon salt
- ½ teaspoon ground ginger
- ¼ teaspoon crushed red pepper flakes
- 1 medium scallion, trimmed and sliced

1. Combine all ingredients in a large bowl. Spoon out 2 tablespoons mixture and roll into a ball. Repeat to form eighteen meatballs total.
2. Place meatballs into ungreased air fryer basket. Adjust the temperature to 400ºF (204ºC) and air fry for 12 minutes, shaking the basket three times throughout cooking. Meatballs will be browned and have an internal temperature of at least 145ºF (63ºC) when done. Serve warm.

Per Serving:calorie: 27 / fat: 2g / protein: 6g / carbs: 0g / sugars: 0g / fiber: 0g / sodium: 54mg

BBQ Ribs and Broccoli Slaw

Prep time: 10 minutes / Cook time: 50 minutes / Serves 6

- BBQ Ribs
- 4 pounds baby back ribs • 1 teaspoon fine sea salt
- 1 teaspoon freshly ground black pepper
- Broccoli Slaw
- ½ cup plain 2 percent Greek yogurt
- 1 tablespoon olive oil
- 1 tablespoon fresh lemon juice
- ½ teaspoon fine sea salt
- ¼ teaspoon freshly ground black pepper
- 1 pound broccoli florets (or florets from 2 large crowns), chopped
- 10 radishes, halved and thinly sliced
- 1 red bell pepper, seeded and cut lengthwise into narrow strips
- 1 large apple (such as Fuji, Jonagold, or Gala), thinly sliced
- ½ red onion, thinly sliced
- ¾ cup low-sugar or unsweetened barbecue sauce

1. To make the ribs: Pat the ribs dry with paper towels, then cut the racks into six sections (three to five ribs per section, depending on how big the racks are). Season the ribs all over with the salt and pepper.
2. Pour 1 cup water into the Instant Pot and place the wire metal steam rack into the pot. Place the ribs on top of the wire rack (it's fine to stack them up).
3. Secure the lid and set the Pressure Release to Sealing. Select the Pressure Cook or Manual setting and set the cooking time for 20 minutes at high pressure. (The pot will take about 15 minutes to come up to pressure before the cooking program begins.)
4. To make the broccoli slaw: While the ribs are cooking, in a small bowl, stir together the yogurt, oil, lemon juice, salt, and pepper, mixing well. In a large bowl, combine the broccoli, radishes, bell pepper, apple, and onion. Drizzle with the yogurt mixture and toss until evenly coated.
5. When the ribs have about 10 minutes left in their cooking time, preheat the oven to 400°F. Line a sheet pan with aluminum foil.
6. When the cooking program ends, perform a quick pressure release by moving the Pressure Release to Venting. Open the pot and, using tongs, transfer the ribs in a single layer to the prepared sheet pan. Brush the barbecue sauce onto both sides of the ribs, using 2 tablespoons of sauce per section of ribs. Bake, meaty-side up, for 15 to 20 minutes, until lightly browned.
7. Serve the ribs warm, with the slaw on the side.

Per Serving:calories: 392 / fat: 15g / protein: 45g / carbs: 19g / sugars: 9g / fiber: 4g / sodium: 961mg

Parmesan-Crusted Pork Chops

Prep time: 5 minutes / Cook time: 12 minutes / Serves 4

- 1 large egg   • ½ cup grated Parmesan cheese
- 4 (4-ounce / 113-g) boneless pork chops
- ½ teaspoon salt • ¼ teaspoon ground black pepper

1. Whisk egg in a medium bowl and place Parmesan in a separate medium bowl.
2. Sprinkle pork chops on both sides with salt and pepper. Dip each pork chop into egg, then press both sides into Parmesan.
3. Place pork chops into ungreased air fryer basket. Adjust the temperature to 400°F (204°C) and air fry for 12 minutes, turning chops halfway through cooking. Pork chops will be golden and have an internal temperature of at least 145°F (63°C) when done. Serve warm.

Per Serving:calorie: 265 / fat: 13g / protein: 32g / carbs: 3g / sugars: 0g / fiber: 0g / sodium: 674mg

Pork Tenderloin Stir-Fry

Prep time: 5 minutes / Cook time: 20 minutes / Serves 6

- 1 tablespoon sesame oil
- 1-pound pork tenderloin, cut into thin strips
- 1 tablespoon oyster sauce (found in the Asian food section of the grocery store)
- 1 tablespoon cornstarch
- ½ cup low-sodium chicken broth
- 1 tablespoon light soy sauce
- 1 cup fresh snow peas, trimmed
- 1 cup broccoli florets
- ½ cup sliced water chestnuts, drained
- 1 cup diced red pepper • ¼ cup sliced scallions

1. In a large skillet or wok, heat the oil. Stir-fry the pork until the strips are no longer pink.
2. In a measuring cup, combine the oyster sauce, cornstarch, chicken broth, and soy sauce. Add the sauce to the pork, and cook until the sauce thickens.
3. Add the vegetables, cover, and steam for 5 minutes. Serve.

Per Serving:calorie: 149 / fat: 5g / protein: 18g / carbs: 8g / sugars: 3g / fiber: 0g / sodium: 174mg

Pork Chops with Raspberry-Chipotle Sauce and Herbed Rice

Prep time: 25 minutes / Cook time: 10 minutes / Serves 4

- Pork Chops
- 4 bone-in pork rib chops, about ¾ inch thick
- ½ teaspoon garlic-pepper blend
- 1 tablespoon canola oil
- Raspberry-Chipotle Sauce
- ⅓ cup all-fruit raspberry spread
- 1 tablespoon water
- 1 tablespoon raspberry-flavored vinegar
- 1 large or 2 small chipotle chiles in adobo sauce,

finely chopped (from 7 ounces can)
- Herbed Rice
- 1 package (8. 8 ounces) quick-cooking (ready in 90 seconds) whole-grain brown rice
- ¼ teaspoon salt-free garlic-herb blend
- ½ teaspoon lemon peel
- 1 tablespoon chopped fresh cilantro

1. Sprinkle pork with garlic pepper. In 12-inch nonstick skillet, heat oil over medium-high heat. Add pork to oil. Cook 8 to 10 minutes, turning once, until pork is no longer pink and meat thermometer inserted in center reads 145°F. Remove from skillet to serving platter (reserve pork drippings); keep warm.
2. Meanwhile, in small bowl, stir raspberry spread, water, vinegar and chile; set aside. Make rice as directed on package. Stir in remaining rice ingredients; keep warm.
3. In skillet with pork drippings, pour raspberry mixture. Cook and stir over low heat about 1 minute or until sauce is bubbly and slightly thickened. Serve pork chops with sauce and rice.

Per Serving:calories: 370 / fat: 12g / protein: 31g / carbs: 34g / sugars: 12g / fiber: 0g / sodium: 140mg

Mustard-Glazed Pork Chops

Prep time: 5 minutes / Cook time: 25 minutes / Serves 4

- ¼ cup Dijon mustard
- 1 tablespoon pure maple syrup
- 2 tablespoons rice vinegar
- 4 bone-in, thin-cut pork chops

1. Preheat the oven to 400°F.
2. In a small saucepan, combine the mustard, maple syrup, and rice vinegar. Stir to mix and bring to a simmer over medium heat. Cook for about 2 minutes until just slightly thickened.
3. In a baking dish, place the pork chops and spoon the sauce over them, flipping to coat.
4. Bake, uncovered, for 18 to 22 minutes until the juices run clear.

Per Serving:calories: 257 / fat: 7g / protein: 39g / carbs: 7g / sugars: 4g / fiber: 0g / sodium: 466mg

Basic Nutritional Values

Prep time: 20 minutes / Cook time: 2 hours / Serves 4 to 6

- 2 pounds beef roast, boneless
- ¼ teaspoon salt   • ¼ teaspoon pepper
- 1 tablespoon olive oil   • 2 stalks celery, chopped
- 4 tablespoons margarine
- 2 cups low-sodium tomato juice
- 2 cloves garlic, finely chopped, or 1 teaspoon garlic powder
- 1 tcaspoon thyme   • 1 bay leaf

- 4 carrots, chopped   • 1 medium onion, chopped
- 4 medium potatoes, chopped

1. Pat beef dry with paper towels; season on all sides with salt and pepper.
2. Select Sauté function on the Instant Pot and adjust heat to more. Put the oil in the inner pot, then cook the beef in oil for 6 minutes, until browned, turning once. Set on plate.
3. Add celery and margarine to the inner pot; cook 2 minutes. Stir in tomato juice, garlic, thyme, and bay leaf. Hit Cancel to turn off Sauté function.
4. Place beef on top of the contents of the inner pot and press into sauce. Cover and lock lid and make sure vent is at sealing. Select Manual and cook at high pressure for 1 hour 15 minutes.
5. Once cooking is complete, release pressure by using natural release function. Transfer beef to cutting board. Discard bay leaf.
6. Skim off any excess fat from surface. Choose Sauté function and adjust heat to more. Cook 18 minutes, or until reduced by about half (2½ cups). Hit Cancel to turn off Sauté function.
7. Add carrots, onion, and potatoes. Cover and lock lid and make sure vent is at sealing. Select Manual and cook at high pressure for 10 minutes.
8. Once cooking is complete, release pressure by using a quick release. Using Sauté function, keep at a simmer.
9. Season with more salt and pepper to taste.

Per Serving:calories: 391 / fat: 19 g / protein: 34g / carbs: 22g / sugars: 6g / fiber: 4g / sodium: 395mg

Steak Stroganoff

Prep time: 15 minutes / Cook time: 30 minutes / Serves 6

- 1 tablespoon olive oil   • 2 tablespoons flour
- ½ teaspoon garlic powder
- ½ teaspoon pepper   • ¼ teaspoon paprika
- 1¾ pounds boneless beef round steak, trimmed of fat, cut into 1½ × ½-inch strips.
- 10¾ ounces can reduced-sodium, 98% fat-free cream of mushroom soup
- ½ cup water
- 1 envelope sodium-free dried onion soup mix
- 9 ounces jar sliced mushrooms, drained
- ½ cup fat-free sour cream
- 1 tablespoon minced fresh parsley

1. Place the oil in the Instant Pot and press Sauté.
2. Combine flour, garlic powder, pepper, and paprika in a small bowl. Stir the steak pieces through the flour mixture until they are evenly coated.
3. Lightly brown the steak pieces in the oil in the Instant Pot, about 2 minutes each side. Press Cancel when done.
4. Stir the mushroom soup, water, and onion soup

mix then pour over the steak.

5. Secure the lid and set the vent to sealing. Press the Manual button and set for 15 minutes.
6. When cook time is up, let the pressure release naturally for 15 minutes, then release the rest manually.
7. Remove the lid and press Cancel then Sauté. Stir in mushrooms, sour cream, and parsley. Let the sauce come to a boil and cook for about 10 to 15 minutes.

Per Serving:calories: 248 / fat: 6g / protein: 33g / carbs: 12g / sugars: 2g / fiber: 2g / sodium: 563mg

Cheeseburger and Cauliflower Wraps

Prep time: 5 minutes / Cook time: 20 minutes / Serves 4

• Avocado oil cooking spray
• ½ cup chopped white onion
• 1 cup chopped portobello mushrooms
• 1 pound 93% lean ground beef
• ½ teaspoon garlic powder   • Pinch salt
• 1 (10-ounce) bag frozen cauliflower rice
• 12 iceberg lettuce leaves
• ¾ cup shredded Cheddar cheese

1. Heat a large skillet over medium heat. When hot, coat the cooking surface with cooking spray and add the onion and mushrooms. Cook for 5 minutes, stirring occasionally.
2. Add the beef, garlic powder, and salt, stirring and breaking apart the meat as needed. Cook for 5 minutes.
3. Stir in the frozen cauliflower rice and increase the heat to medium-high. Cook for 5 minutes more, or until the water evaporates.
4. For each portion, use three lettuce leaves. Spoon one-quarter of the filling onto the lettuce leaves, and top with one-quarter of the cheese. Then, working from the side closest to you, roll up the lettuce to close the wrap. Repeat with the remaining lettuce leaves and filling.

Per Serving:calorie: 274 / fat: 13g / protein: 32g / carbs: 8g / sugars: 4g / fiber: 3g / sodium: 242mg

Mexican-Style Shredded Beef

Prep time: 5 minutes / Cook time: 35 minutes / Serves 6

• 1 (2-pound / 907-g) beef chuck roast, cut into 2-inch cubes   • 1 teaspoon salt
• ½ teaspoon ground black pepper
• ½ cup no-sugar-added chipotle sauce

1. In a large bowl, sprinkle beef cubes with salt and pepper and toss to coat. Place beef into ungreased air fryer basket. Adjust the temperature to 400°F (204°C) and air fry for 30 minutes, shaking the basket halfway through cooking. Beef will be done when internal temperature is at least 160°F

(71°C).
2. Place cooked beef into a large bowl and shred with two forks. Pour in chipotle sauce and toss to coat.
3. Return beef to air fryer basket for an additional 5 minutes at 400°F (204°C) to crisp with sauce. Serve warm.

Per Serving:calorie: 295 / fat: 16g / protein: 31g / carbs: 3g / sugars: 2g / fiber: 0g / sodium: 449mg

Grilled Pork Loin Chops

Prep time: 15 minutes / Cook time: 30 minutes / Serves 2

• 2 garlic cloves, minced
• 3 tablespoons Worcestershire sauce
• 2 tablespoons water
• 1 tablespoon low-sodium soy sauce
• 2 teaspoons tomato paste
• 1 teaspoon granulated stevia
• ½ teaspoon ground ginger
• ½ teaspoon onion powder
• ¼ teaspoon cinnamon
• ⅛ teaspoon cayenne pepper
• 2 (6 ounces) thick-cut boneless pork loin chops
• Olive oil, for greasing the grill

1. In a small bowl, mix together the garlic, Worcestershire sauce, water, soy sauce, tomato paste, stevia, ginger, onion powder, cinnamon, and cayenne pepper. Pour half of the marinade into a large plastic sealable bag. Cover and refrigerate the remaining marinade.
2. Add the pork chops to the bag and seal. Refrigerate for 4 to 8 hours, turning occasionally.
3. Preheat the grill to medium.
4. With the olive oil, lightly oil the grill grate.
5. Remove the pork chops from the bag. Discard the marinade in the bag.
6. Place the chops on the preheated grill, basting with the remaining reserved half of the marinade. Grill for 8 to 12 minutes per side, or until the meat is browned, no longer pink inside, and an instant-read thermometer inserted into the thickest part of the chop reads at least 145°F.
7. In a saucepan set over medium heat, pour any remaining reserved marinade. Bring to a boil. Reduce the heat to low. Simmer for about 5 minutes, stirring constantly, until slightly thickened.
8. To serve, plate the chops and spoon the sauce over.

Per Serving:calorie: 254 / fat: 6g / protein: 39g / carbs: 9g / sugars: 3g / fiber: 1g / sodium: 593mg

Beef Burrito Bowl

Prep time: 5 minutes / Cook time: 15 minutes / Serves 4

• 1 pound 93% lean ground beef
• 1 cup canned low-sodium black beans, drained and

rinsed
- ¼ teaspoon ground cumin
- ¼ teaspoon chili powder
- ¼ teaspoon garlic powder
- ¼ teaspoon onion powder
- ¼ teaspoon salt
- 1 head romaine or preferred lettuce, shredded
- 2 medium tomatoes, chopped
- 1 cup shredded Cheddar cheese or packaged cheese blend

1. Heat a large skillet over medium-low heat. Put the beef, beans, cumin, chili powder, garlic powder, onion powder, and salt into the skillet, and cook for 8 to 10 minutes, until cooked through. Stir occasionally.
2. Divide the lettuce evenly between four bowls. Add one-quarter of the beef mixture to each bowl and top with one-quarter of the tomatoes and cheese.

Per Serving:calorie: 358 / fat: 16g / protein: 37g / carbs: 18g / sugars: 4g / fiber: 8g / sodium: 506mg

Pork Milanese

Prep time: 10 minutes / Cook time: 12 minutes / Serves 4

- 4 (1-inch) boneless pork chops
- Fine sea salt and ground black pepper, to taste
- 2 large eggs • ¾ cup powdered Parmesan cheese
- Chopped fresh parsley, for garnish
- Lemon slices, for serving

1. Spray the air fryer basket with avocado oil. Preheat the air fryer to 400ºF (204ºC).
2. Place the pork chops between 2 sheets of plastic wrap and pound them with the flat side of a meat tenderizer until they're ¼ inch thick. Lightly season both sides of the chops with salt and pepper.
3. Lightly beat the eggs in a shallow bowl. Divide the Parmesan cheese evenly between 2 bowls and set the bowls in this order: Parmesan, eggs, Parmesan. Dredge a chop in the first bowl of Parmesan, then dip it in the eggs, and then dredge it again in the second bowl of Parmesan, making sure both sides and all edges are well coated. Repeat with the remaining chops.
4. Place the chops in the air fryer basket and air fry for 12 minutes, or until the internal temperature reaches 145ºF (63ºC), flipping halfway through.
5. Garnish with fresh parsley and serve immediately with lemon slices. Store leftovers in an airtight container in the refrigerator for up to 3 days. Reheat in a preheated 390ºF (199ºC) air fryer for 5 minutes, or until warmed through.

Per Serving:calorie: 370 / fat: 21g / protein: 39g / carbs: 4g / sugars: 0g / fiber: 0g / sodium: 660mg

Beef Burgundy

Prep time: 30 minutes / Cook time: 30 minutes / Serves 6

- 2 tablespoons olive oil
- 2 pounds stewing meat, cubed, trimmed of fat
- 2½ tablespoons flour
- 5 medium onions, thinly sliced
- ½ pound fresh mushrooms, sliced
- 1 teaspoon salt • ¼ teaspoon dried marjoram
- ¼ teaspoon dried thyme
- ⅛ teaspoon pepper   • ¾ cup beef broth
- 1½ cups burgundy

1. Press Sauté on the Instant pot and add in the olive oil.
2. Dredge meat in flour, then brown in batches in the Instant Pot. Set aside the meat. Sauté the onions and mushrooms in the remaining oil and drippings for about 3–4 minutes, then add the meat back in. Press Cancel.
3. Add the salt, marjoram, thyme, pepper, broth, and wine to the Instant Pot.
4. Secure the lid and make sure the vent is set to sealing. Press the Manual button and set to 30 minutes.
5. When cook time is up, let the pressure release naturally for 15 minutes, then perform a quick release.
6. Serve over cooked noodles.

Per Serving:calories: 358 / fat: 11g / protein: 37g / carbs: 15g / sugars: 5g / fiber: 2g / sodium: 472mg

Spiced Lamb Stew

Prep time: 20 minutes / Cook time: 2 hours / Serves 4

- 2 tablespoons extra-virgin olive oil
- 1½ pounds lamb shoulder, cut into 1-inch chunks
- ½ sweet onion, chopped
- 1 tablespoon grated fresh ginger
- 2 teaspoons minced garlic
- 1 teaspoon ground cinnamon
- 1 teaspoon ground cumin
- ¼ teaspoon ground cloves
- 2 sweet potatoes, peeled, diced
- 2 cups low-sodium beef broth
- Sea salt
- Freshly ground back pepper
- 2 teaspoons chopped fresh parsley, for garnish

1. Preheat the oven to 300ºF.
2. Place a large ovenproof skillet over medium-high heat and add the olive oil.
3. Brown the lamb, stirring occasionally, for about 6 minutes.
4. Add the onion, ginger, garlic, cinnamon, cumin, and cloves, and sauté for 5 minutes.
5. Add the sweet potatoes and beef broth and bring the stew to a boil.
6. Cover the skillet and transfer the lamb to the oven. Braise, stirring occasionally, until the lamb is very

tender, about 2 hours.

7. Remove the stew from the oven and season with salt and pepper.
8. Serve garnished with the parsley.

*Per Serving:*calorie: 406 / fat: 21g / protein: 37g / carbs: 18g / sugars: 5g / fiber: 3g / sodium: 511mg

Homestyle Herb Meatballs

Prep time: 10 minutes / Cook time: 15 minutes / Serves 4

- ½ pound lean ground pork
- ½ pound lean ground beef
- 1 sweet onion, finely chopped
- ¼ cup bread crumbs
- 2 tablespoons chopped fresh basil
- 2 teaspoons minced garlic
- 1 egg   • Pinch sea salt
- Pinch freshly ground black pepper

1. Preheat the oven to 350°F.
2. Line a baking tray with parchment paper and set it aside.
3. In a large bowl, mix together the pork, beef, onion, bread crumbs, basil, garlic, egg, salt, and pepper until very well mixed.
4. Roll the meat mixture into 2-inch meatballs.
5. Transfer the meatballs to the baking sheet and bake until they are browned and cooked through, about 15 minutes.
6. Serve the meatballs with your favorite marinara sauce and some steamed green beans.

*Per Serving:*calorie: 214 / fat: 7g / protein: 27g / carbs: 12g / sugars: 5g / fiber: 1g / sodium: 147mg

Smothered Sirloin

Prep time: 15 minutes / Cook time: 30 minutes / Serves 5

- 1 pound beef round sirloin tip
- 1 teaspoon freshly ground black pepper
- 1 teaspoon celery seeds
- 2 tablespoons extra-virgin olive oil
- 1 medium yellow onion, chopped
- ¼ cup chickpea flour
- 2 cups store-bought low-sodium chicken broth, divided
- 2 celery stalks, thinly sliced
- 1 medium red bell pepper, chopped
- 2 garlic cloves, minced
- 2 tablespoons whole-wheat flour
- Generous pinch cayenne pepper
- Chopped fresh chives, for garnish (optional)
- Smoked paprika, for garnish (optional)

1. In a bowl, season the steak on both sides with the black pepper and celery seeds.
2. Select the Sauté setting on an electric pressure cooker, and combine the olive oil and onions. Cook for 3 to 5 minutes, stirring, or until the

onions are browned but not burned.

3. Slowly add the chickpea flour, 1 tablespoon at a time, while stirring.
4. Add 1 cup of broth, ¼ cup at a time, as needed.
5. Stir in the celery, bell pepper, and garlic and cook for 3 to 5 minutes, or until softened.
6. Lay the beef on top of vegetables, and pour the remaining 1 cup of broth on top.
7. Close and lock the lid and set the pressure valve to sealing.
8. Change to the Manual/Pressure Cook setting, and cook for 20 minutes.
9. Once cooking is complete, quick-release the pressure. Carefully remove the lid.
10. Remove the steak and vegetables from the pressure cooker, reserving the leftover liquid for the gravy base.
11. To make the gravy, add the whole-wheat flour and cayenne to the liquid in the pressure cooker, mixing continuously until thickened.
12. To serve, spoon the gravy over the steak and garnish with the chives (if using) and paprika (if using).

*Per Serving:*calorie: 234 / fat: 11g / protein: 23g / carbs: 11g / sugars: 3g / fiber: 2g / sodium: 96mg

Open-Faced Philly Cheesesteak Sandwiches

Prep time: 5 minutes / Cook time: 25 minutes / Serves 4

- Avocado oil cooking spray
- 1 cup chopped yellow onion
- 1 green bell pepper, chopped
- 12 ounces 93% lean ground beef
- Pinch salt
- ¾ teaspoon freshly ground black pepper
- 4 slices provolone or Swiss cheese
- 4 English muffins, 100% whole-wheat

1. Heat a large skillet over medium-low heat. When hot, coat the cooking surface with cooking spray, and arrange the onion and pepper in an even layer. Cook for 8 to 10 minutes, stirring every 3 to 4 minutes.
2. Push the vegetables to one side of the skillet and add the beef, breaking it into large chunks. Cook for 7 to 9 minutes, until a crisp crust forms on the bottom of the meat.
3. Season the beef with the salt and pepper, then flip the beef over and break it down into smaller chunks.
4. Stir the vegetables and the beef together, then top with the cheese and cook for 2 minutes.
5. Meanwhile, split each muffin in half, if necessary, then toast the muffins in a toaster.
6. Place one-eighth of the filling on each muffin half.

*Per Serving:*calorie: 373 / fat: 13g / protein: 33g / carbs: 33g / sugars: 8g / fiber: 6g / sodium: 303mg

Apple Cinnamon Pork Chops

Prep time: 5 minutes / Cook time: 20 minutes / Serves 2

- 2 teaspoons extra-virgin olive oil
- 1 large apple, sliced
- ½ teaspoon organic cinnamon
- ⅛ teaspoon freshly grated nutmeg
- Two 3-ounce lean boneless pork chops, trimmed of fat

1. In a medium nonstick skillet, heat the olive oil. Add the apple slices, and sauté until just tender. Sprinkle with cinnamon and nutmeg, remove from heat, and keep warm.
2. Place the pork chops in the skillet, and cook thoroughly; a meat thermometer inserted into the thickest part of the meat should reach 145 degrees. Remove the pork chops from the skillet, arrange on a serving platter, spoon the apple slices on top, and serve.

Per Serving:calorie: 208 / fat: 8g / protein: 19g / carbs: 16g / sugars: 11g / fiber: 3g / sodium: 43mg

Roasted Pork Loin

Prep time: 5 minutes / Cook time: 40 minutes / Serves 4

- 1 pound pork loin
- 1 tablespoon extra-virgin olive oil, divided
- 2 teaspoons honey
- ¼ teaspoon freshly ground black pepper
- ½ teaspoon dried rosemary
- 2 small gold potatoes, chopped into 2-inch cubes
- 4 (6-inch) carrots, chopped into ½-inch rounds

1. Preheat the oven to 350ºF.
2. Rub the pork loin with ½ tablespoon of oil and the honey. Season with the pepper and rosemary.
3. In a medium bowl, toss the potatoes and carrots in the remaining ½ tablespoon of oil.
4. Place the pork and the vegetables on a baking sheet in a single layer. Cook for 40 minutes.
5. Remove the baking sheet from the oven and let the pork rest for at least 10 minutes before slicing. Divide the pork and vegetables into four equal portions.

Per Serving:calorie: 281 / fat: 8g / protein: 28g / carbs: 24g / sugars: 6g / fiber: 4g / sodium: 103mg

Red Wine Pot Roast with Winter Vegetables

Prep time: 10 minutes / Cook time: 1 hour 35 minutes / Serves 6

- One 3-pound boneless beef chuck roast or bottom round roast (see Note)
- 2 teaspoons fine sea salt
- 1 teaspoon freshly ground black pepper
- 1 tablespoon cold-pressed avocado oil
- 4 large shallots, quartered
- 4 garlic cloves, minced
- 1 cup dry red wine
- 2 tablespoons Dijon mustard
- 2 teaspoons chopped fresh rosemary
- 1 pound parsnips or turnips, cut into ½-inch pieces
- 1 pound carrots, cut into ½-inch pieces
- 4 celery stalks, cut into ½-inch pieces

1. Put the beef onto a plate, pat it dry with paper towels, and then season all over with the salt and pepper.
2. Select the Sauté setting on the Instant Pot and heat the oil for 2 minutes. Using tongs, lower the roast into the pot and sear for about 4 minutes, until browned on the first side. Flip the roast and sear for about 4 minutes more, until browned on the second side. Return the roast to the plate.
3. Add the shallots to the pot and sauté for about 2 minutes, until they begin to soften. Add the garlic and sauté for about 1 minute more. Stir in the wine, mustard, and rosemary, using a wooden spoon to nudge any browned bits from the bottom of the pot. Return the roast to the pot, then spoon some of the cooking liquid over the top.
4. Secure the lid and set the Pressure Release to Sealing. Press the Cancel button to reset the cooking program, then select the Meat/Stew setting and set the cooking time for 1 hour 5 minutes at high pressure. (The pot will take about 5 minutes to come up to pressure before the cooking program begins.)
5. When the cooking program ends, let the pressure release naturally for at least 15 minutes, then move the Pressure Release to Venting to release any remaining steam. Open the pot and, using tongs, carefully transfer the pot roast to a cutting board. Tent with aluminum foil to keep warm.
6. Add the parsnips, carrots, and celery to the pot.
7. Secure the lid and set the Pressure Release to Sealing. Press the Cancel button to reset the cooking program, then select the Pressure Cook or Manual setting and set the cooking time for 3 minutes at low pressure. (The pot will take about 10 minutes to come up to pressure before the cooking program begins.)
8. When the cooking program ends, perform a quick pressure release by moving the Pressure Release to Venting. Open the pot and, using a slotted spoon, transfer the vegetables to a serving dish. Wearing heat-resistant mitts, lift out the inner pot and pour the cooking liquid into a gravy boat or other serving vessel with a spout. (If you like, use a fat separator to remove the fat from the liquid before serving.)
9. If the roast was tied, snip the string and discard.

Carve the roast against the grain into ½-inch-thick slices and arrange them on the dish with the vegetables. Pour some cooking liquid over the roast and serve, passing the remaining cooking liquid on the side.

Per Serving:calorie: 448 / fat: 25g / protein: 26g / carbs: 26g / sugars: 7g / fiber: 6g / sodium: 945mg

Sage-Parmesan Pork Chops

Prep time: 30 minutes / Cook time: 25 minutes / Serves 2

- Extra-virgin olive oil cooking spray
- 2 tablespoons coconut flour
- ¼ teaspoon salt
- Pinch freshly ground black pepper
- ¼ cup almond meal
- ½ cup finely ground flaxseed meal
- ½ cup soy Parmesan cheese
- 1½ teaspoons rubbed sage
- ½ teaspoon grated lemon zest
- 2 (4-ounce) boneless pork chops
- 1 large egg, lightly beaten
- 1 tablespoon extra-virgin olive oil

1. Preheat the oven to 425°F.
2. Lightly coat a medium baking dish with cooking spray.
3. In a shallow dish, mix together the coconut flour, salt, and pepper.
4. In a second shallow dish, stir together the almond meal, flaxseed meal, soy Parmesan cheese, sage, and lemon zest.
5. Gently press one pork chop into the coconut flour mixture to coat. Shake off any excess. Dip into the beaten egg. Press into the almond meal mixture. Gently toss between your hands so any coating that hasn't stuck can fall away. Place the coated chop on a plate. Repeat the process with the remaining pork chop and coating ingredients.
6. In a large skillet set over medium heat, heat the olive oil.
7. Add the coated chops. Cook for about 4 minutes per side, or until browned. Transfer to the prepared baking dish. Place the dish in the preheated oven. Bake for 10 to 15 minutes, or until the juices run clear and an instant-read thermometer inserted into the middle of the pork reads 160°F.

Per Serving:calorie: 520 / fat: 31g / protein: 45g / carbs: 14g / sugars: 1g / fiber: 6g / sodium: 403mg

Pork Chops Pomodoro

Prep time: 0 minutes / Cook time: 30 minutes / Serves 6

- 2 pounds boneless pork loin chops, each about 5⅓ ounces and ½ inch thick
- ¾ teaspoon fine sea salt
- ½ teaspoon freshly ground black pepper
- 2 tablespoons extra-virgin olive oil
- 2 garlic cloves, chopped
- ½ cup low-sodium chicken broth or vegetable broth
- ½ teaspoon Italian seasoning
- 1 tablespoon capers, drained
- 2 cups cherry tomatoes
- 2 tablespoons chopped fresh basil or flat-leaf parsley
- Spiralized zucchini noodles, cooked cauliflower "rice," or cooked whole-grain pasta for serving
- Lemon wedges for serving

1. Pat the pork chops dry with paper towels, then season them all over with the salt and pepper.
2. Select the Sauté setting on the Instant Pot and heat 1 tablespoon of the oil for 2 minutes. Swirl the oil to coat the bottom of the pot. Using tongs, add half of the pork chops in a single layer and sear for about 3 minutes, until lightly browned on the first side. Flip the chops and sear for about 3 minutes more, until lightly browned on the second side. Transfer the chops to a plate. Repeat with the remaining 1 tablespoon oil and pork chops.
3. Add the garlic to the pot and sauté for about 1 minute, until bubbling but not browned. Stir in the broth, Italian seasoning, and capers, using a wooden spoon to nudge any browned bits from the bottom of the pot and working quickly so not too much liquid evaporates. Using the tongs, transfer the pork chops to the pot. Add the tomatoes in an even layer on top of the chops.
4. Secure the lid and set the Pressure Release to Sealing. Press the Cancel button to reset the cooking program, then select the Pressure Cook or Manual setting and set the cooking time for 10 minutes at high pressure. (The pot will take about 5 minutes to come up to pressure before the cooking program begins.)
5. When the cooking program ends, let the pressure release naturally for at least 10 minutes, then move the Pressure Release to Venting to release any remaining steam. Open the pot and, using the tongs, transfer the pork chops to a serving dish.
6. Spoon the tomatoes and some of the cooking liquid on top of the pork chops. Sprinkle with the basil and serve right away, with zucchini noodles and lemon wedges on the side.

Per Serving:calorie: 265 / fat: 13g / protein: 31g / carbs: 3g / sugars: 2g / fiber: 1g / sodium: 460mg

Chapter 5 Fish and Seafood

Ahi Tuna Steaks

Prep time: 5 minutes / Cook time: 14 minutes / Serves 2

- 2 (6 ounces / 170 g) ahi tuna steaks
- 2 tablespoons olive oil
- 3 tablespoons everything bagel seasoning

1. Drizzle both sides of each steak with olive oil. Place seasoning on a medium plate and press each side of tuna steaks into seasoning to form a thick layer.
2. Place steaks into ungreased air fryer basket. Adjust the temperature to 400ºF (204ºC) and air fry for 14 minutes, turning steaks halfway through cooking. Steaks will be done when internal temperature is at least 145ºF (63ºC) for well-done. Serve warm.

Per Serving:calorie: 400 / fat: 24g / protein: 40g / carbs: 4g / sugars: 0g / fiber: 2g / sodium: 600mg

Halibut with Lime and Cilantro

Prep time: 30 minutes / Cook time: 10 to 20 minutes / Serves 2

- 2 tablespoons lime juice
- 1 tablespoon chopped fresh cilantro
- 1 teaspoon olive or canola oil
- 1 clove garlic, finely chopped
- 2 halibut or salmon steaks (about ¾ pound)
- Freshly ground pepper to taste
- ½ cup chunky-style salsa

1. In shallow glass or plastic dish or in resealable food-storage plastic bag, mix lime juice, cilantro, oil and garlic. Add halibut, turning several times to coat with marinade. Cover; refrigerate 15 minutes, turning once.
2. Heat gas or charcoal grill. Remove halibut from marinade; discard marinade.
3. Place halibut on grill over medium heat. Cover grill; cook 10 to 20 minutes, turning once, until halibut flakes easily with fork. Sprinkle with pepper. Serve with salsa.

Per Serving:calories: 190 / fat: 4. 5g / protein: 32g / carbs: 6g / sugars: 2g / fiber: 0g / sodium: 600mg

Walnut-Crusted Halibut with Pear Salad

Prep time: 10 minutes / Cook time: 10 minutes / Serves 4

- For the halibut
- ¾ cup finely chopped toasted walnuts
- 2 tablespoons bread crumbs
- ¼ cup chopped fresh parsley
- 2 tablespoons chopped fresh chives

- 4 (6 to 8 ounces) halibut fillets
- Kosher salt
- Freshly ground black pepper
- 1 tablespoon extra-virgin olive oil
- For the salad
- 6 cups packed mixed greens
- 1 pear, thinly sliced
- ¼ cup chopped fresh parsley
- ¼ cup chopped fresh chives
- Zest and juice of 1 lemon
- Extra-virgin olive oil, for the dressing
- Kosher salt
- Freshly ground black pepper

To make the halibut 1. Preheat the broiler. Line a baking sheet with parchment paper.
2. In a small bowl, combine the walnuts, bread crumbs, parsley, and chives.
3. Pat the halibut fillets dry, season them with salt and pepper and rub ½ tablespoon of extra-virgin olive oil on each fillet. Place the fillets on the prepared baking sheet. Sprinkle the walnut mixture evenly on top of each fillet and press slightly, so the topping will stick.
4. Broil the fish until the crust is golden and the fish is fully cooked, 5 to 8 minutes. To make the salad
5. Meanwhile, in a large bowl, toss the greens, pear, parsley, chives, and zest until well combined. Drizzle the salad with the lemon juice and a bit of extra-virgin olive oil to taste. Season with salt and pepper to taste.
6. Evenly divide the salad among four plates and top with the fish. Serve.
7. Store any leftovers in an airtight container in the refrigerator for up to 2 days.

Per Serving:calories: 551 / fat: 43g / protein: 31g / carbs: 13g / sugars: 4g / fiber: 5g / sodium: 196mg

Ginger-Garlic Cod Cooked in Paper

Prep time: 10 minutes / Cook time: 15 minutes / Serves 4

- 1 chard bunch, stemmed, leaves and stems cut into thin strips
- 1 red bell pepper, seeded and cut into strips
- 1 pound cod fillets cut into 4 pieces
- 1 tablespoon grated fresh ginger
- 3 garlic cloves, minced
- 2 tablespoons white wine vinegar
- 2 tablespoons low-sodium tamari or gluten-free soy sauce
- 1 tablespoon honey

1. Preheat the oven to 425°F.

2. Cut four pieces of parchment paper, each about 16 inches wide. Lay the four pieces out on a large workspace.
3. On each piece of paper, arrange a small pile of chard leaves and stems, topped by several strips of bell pepper. Top with a piece of cod.
4. In a small bowl, mix the ginger, garlic, vinegar, tamari, and honey. Top each piece of fish with one-fourth of the mixture.
5. Fold the parchment paper over so the edges overlap. Fold the edges over several times to secure the fish in the packets. Carefully place the packets on a large baking sheet.
6. Bake for 12 minutes. Carefully open the packets, allowing steam to escape, and serve.

Per Serving:calories: 118 / fat: 1g / protein: 19g / carbs: 9g / sugars: 6g / fiber: 1g / sodium: 715mg

Cobia with Lemon-Caper Sauce

Prep time: 25 minutes / Cook time: 10 minutes / Serves 4

- ⅓ cup all-purpose flour
- ¼ teaspoon salt
- ¼ teaspoon pepper
- 1¼ lb cobia or sea bass fillets, cut into 4 pieces
- 2 tablespoons olive oil
- ⅓ cup dry white wine
- ½ cup reduced-sodium chicken broth
- 2 tablespoons lemon juice
- 1 tablespoon capers, rinsed, drained
- 1 tablespoon chopped fresh parsley

1. In shallow dish, stir flour, salt and pepper. Coat cobia pieces in flour mixture (reserve remaining flour mixture). In 12-inch nonstick skillet, heat oil over medium-high heat. Place coated cobia in oil. Cook 8 to 10 minutes, turning halfway through cooking, until fish flakes easily with fork; remove from heat. Lift fish from skillet to serving platter with slotted spatula (do not discard drippings); keep warm.
2. Heat skillet (with drippings) over medium heat. Stir in 1 tablespoon reserved flour mixture; cook and stir 30 seconds. Stir in wine; cook about 30 seconds or until thickened and slightly reduced. Stir in chicken broth and lemon juice; cook and stir 1 to 2 minutes until sauce is smooth and slightly thickened. Stir in capers.
3. Serve sauce over cobia; sprinkle with parsley.

Per Serving:calories: 230 / fat: 9g / protein: 28g / carbs: 9g / sugars: 0g / fiber: 0g / sodium: 400mg

Salmon Fritters with Zucchini

Prep time: 15 minutes / Cook time: 12 minutes / Serves 4

- 2 tablespoons almond flour
- 1 zucchini, grated
- 1 egg, beaten
- 6 ounces (170 g) salmon fillet, diced
- 1 teaspoon avocado oil
- ½ teaspoon ground black pepper

1. Mix almond flour with zucchini, egg, salmon, and ground black pepper.
2. Then make the fritters from the salmon mixture.
3. Sprinkle the air fryer basket with avocado oil and put the fritters inside.
4. Cook the fritters at 375°F (191°C) for 6 minutes per side.

Per Serving:calorie: 150 / fat: 9g / protein: 12g / carbs: 4g / sugars: 1g / fiber: 1g / sodium: 70mg

Grilled Rosemary Swordfish

Prep time: 5 minutes / Cook time: 15 minutes / Serves 4

- 2 scallions, thinly sliced
- 2 tablespoons extra-virgin olive oil
- 2 tablespoons white wine vinegar
- 1 teaspoon fresh rosemary, finely chopped
- 4 swordfish steaks (1 pound total)

1. In a small bowl, combine the scallions, olive oil, vinegar, and rosemary. Pour over the swordfish steaks. Let the steaks marinate for 30 minutes.
2. Remove the steaks from the marinade, and grill for 5–7 minutes per side, brushing with marinade. Transfer to a serving platter, and serve.

Per Serving:calories: 225 / fat: 14g / protein: 22g / carbs: 0g / sugars: 0g / fiber: 0g / sodium: 92mg

Baked Salmon with Lemon Sauce

Prep time: 10 minutes / Cook time: 15 minutes / Serves 4

- 4 (5-ounce) salmon fillets
- Sea salt
- Freshly ground black pepper
- 1 tablespoon extra-virgin olive oil
- ½ cup low-sodium vegetable broth
- Juice and zest of 1 lemon
- 1 teaspoon chopped fresh thyme
- ½ cup fat-free sour cream
- 1 teaspoon honey
- 1 tablespoon chopped fresh chives

1. Preheat the oven to 400°F.
2. Season the salmon lightly on both sides with salt and pepper.
3. Place a large ovenproof skillet over medium-high heat and add the olive oil.
4. Sear the salmon fillets on both sides until golden, about 3 minutes per side.
5. Transfer the salmon to a baking dish and bake until it is just cooked through, about 10 minutes.

6. While the salmon is baking, whisk together the vegetable broth, lemon juice, zest, and thyme in a small saucepan over medium-high heat until the liquid reduces by about one-quarter, about 5 minutes.
7. Whisk in the sour cream and honey.
8. Stir in the chives and serve the sauce over the salmon.

Per Serving: calories: 243 / fat: 10g / protein: 30g / carbs: 8g / sugars: 2g / fiber: 1g / sodium: 216mg

Salmon Florentine

Prep time: 10 minutes / Cook time: 30 minutes / Serves 4

- 1 teaspoon extra-virgin olive oil
- ½ sweet onion, finely chopped
- 1 teaspoon minced garlic
- 3 cups baby spinach
- 1 cup kale, tough stems removed, torn into 3-inch pieces
- Sea salt
- Freshly ground black pepper
- 4 (5-ounce) salmon fillets
- Lemon wedges, for serving

1. Preheat the oven to 350°F.
2. Place a large skillet over medium-high heat and add the oil.
3. Sauté the onion and garlic until softened and translucent, about 3 minutes.
4. Add the spinach and kale and sauté until the greens wilt, about 5 minutes.
5. Remove the skillet from the heat and season the greens with salt and pepper.
6. Place the salmon fillets so they are nestled in the greens and partially covered by them. Bake the salmon until it is opaque, about 20 minutes.
7. Serve immediately with a squeeze of fresh lemon.

Per Serving: calories: 211 / fat: 8g / protein: 30g / carbs: 5g / sugars: 2g / fiber: 1g / sodium: 129mg

Shrimp Louie Salad with Thousand Island Dressing

Prep time: 5 minutes / Cook time: 20 minutes / Serves 4

- 2 cups water
- 1½ teaspoons fine sea salt
- 1 pound medium shrimp, peeled and deveined
- 4 large eggs
- Thousand island Dressing
- ¼ cup no-sugar-added ketchup
- ¼ cup mayonnaise
- 1 tablespoon fresh lemon juice
- 1 teaspoon Worcestershire sauce
- ⅛ teaspoon cayenne pepper
- Freshly ground black pepper

- 2 green onions, white and green parts, sliced thinly
- 2 hearts romaine lettuce or 1 head iceberg lettuce, shredded
- 1 English cucumber, sliced
- 8 radishes, sliced
- 1 cup cherry tomatoes, sliced
- 1 large avocado, pitted, peeled, and sliced

1. Combine the water and salt in the Instant Pot and stir to dissolve the salt.
2. Secure the lid and set the Pressure Release to Sealing. Select the Steam setting and set the cooking time for 0 (zero) minutes at low pressure. (The pot will take about 10 minutes to come up to pressure before the cooking program begins.)
3. Meanwhile, prepare an ice bath.
4. When the cooking program ends, perform a quick release by moving the Pressure Release to Venting. Open the pot and stir in the shrimp, using a wooden spoon to nudge them all down into the water. Cover the pot and leave the shrimp for 2 minutes on the Keep Warm setting. The shrimp will gently poach and cook through. Uncover the pot and, wearing heat-resistant mitts, lift out the inner pot and drain the shrimp in a colander. Transfer them to the ice bath to cool for 5 minutes, then drain them in the colander and set aside in the refrigerator.
5. Rinse out the inner pot and return it to the housing. Pour in 1 cup water and place the wire metal steam rack into the pot. Place the eggs on top of the steam rack.
6. Secure the lid and set the Pressure Release to Sealing. Press the Cancel button to reset the cooking program, then select the Egg, Pressure Cook, or Manual setting and set the cooking time for 5 minutes at high pressure. (The pot will take about 5 minutes to come up to pressure before the cooking program begins.)
7. While the eggs are cooking, prepare another ice bath.
8. When the cooking program ends, let the pressure release naturally for 5 minutes, then move the Pressure Release to Venting to release any remaining steam. Using tongs, transfer the eggs to the ice bath and let cool for 5 minutes.
9. To make the dressing: In a small bowl, stir together the ketchup, mayonnaise, lemon juice, Worcestershire sauce, cayenne, ¼ teaspoon black pepper, and green onions.
10. Arrange the lettuce, cucumber, radishes, tomatoes, and avocado on individual plates or in large, shallow individual bowls. Mound the cooked shrimp in the center of each salad. Peel the eggs, quarter them lengthwise, and place the quarters around the shrimp.

11. Spoon the dressing over the salads and top with additional black pepper. Serve right away.

Per Serving:calories: 407 / fat: 23g / protein: 35g / carbs: 16g / sugars: 10g / fiber: 6g / sodium: 1099mg

Spicy Citrus Sole

Prep time: 10 minutes / Cook time: 10 minutes / Serves 4

- 1 teaspoon chili powder
- 1 teaspoon garlic powder
- ½ teaspoon lime zest
- ½ teaspoon lemon zest
- ¼ teaspoon freshly ground black pepper
- ¼ teaspoon smoked paprika
- Pinch sea salt
- 4 (6-ounce) sole fillets, patted dry
- 1 tablespoon extra-virgin olive oil
- 2 teaspoons freshly squeezed lime juice

1. Preheat the oven to 450°F.
2. Line a baking sheet with aluminum foil and set it aside.
3. In a small bowl, stir together the chili powder, garlic powder, lime zest, lemon zest, pepper, paprika, and salt until well mixed.
4. Pat the fish fillets dry with paper towels, place them on the baking sheet, and rub them lightly all over with the spice mixture.
5. Drizzle the olive oil and lime juice on the top of the fish.
6. Bake until the fish flakes when pressed lightly with a fork, about 8 minutes. Serve immediately.

Per Serving:calories: 155 / fat: 7g / protein: 21g / carbs: 1g / sugars: 0g / fiber: 1g / sodium: 524mg

Pecan-Crusted Catfish

Prep time: 5 minutes / Cook time: 12 minutes / Serves 4

- ½ cup pecan meal
- 1 teaspoon fine sea salt
- ¼ teaspoon ground black pepper
- 4 (4 ounces / 113 g) catfish fillets
- For Garnish (Optional):
- Fresh oregano
- Pecan halves

1. Spray the air fryer basket with avocado oil. Preheat the air fryer to 375°F (191°C).
2. In a large bowl, mix the pecan meal, salt, and pepper. One at a time, dredge the catfish fillets in the mixture, coating them well. Use your hands to press the pecan meal into the fillets. Spray the fish with avocado oil and place them in the air fryer basket.
3. Air fry the coated catfish for 12 minutes, or until it flakes easily and is no longer translucent in the center, flipping halfway through.
4. Garnish with oregano sprigs and pecan halves, if desired.
5. Store leftovers in an airtight container in the fridge for up to 3 days. Reheat in a preheated 350°F (177°C) air fryer for 4 minutes, or until heated through.

Per Serving:calorie: 350 / fat: 28g / protein: 20g / carbs: 8g / sugars: 2g / fiber: 4g / sodium: 600mg

Bacon-Wrapped Scallops

Prep time: 5 minutes / Cook time: 10 minutes / Serves 4

- 8 (1-ounce / 28-g) sea scallops, cleaned and patted dry
- 8 slices sugar-free bacon
- ¼ teaspoon salt
- ¼ teaspoon ground black pepper

1. Wrap each scallop in 1 slice bacon and secure with a toothpick. Sprinkle with salt and pepper.
2. Place scallops into ungreased air fryer basket. Adjust the temperature to 360°F (182°C) and air fry for 10 minutes. Scallops will be opaque and firm, and have an internal temperature of 135°F (57°C) when done. Serve warm.

Per Serving:calories: 251 / fat: 21g / protein: 13g / carbs: 2g / sugars: 0g / fiber: 0g / sodium: 612mg

Scallops and Asparagus Skillet

Prep time: 10 minutes / Cook time: 15 minutes / Serves 4

- 3 teaspoons extra-virgin olive oil, divided
- 1 pound asparagus, trimmed and cut into 2-inch segments
- 1 tablespoon butter
- 1 pound sea scallops
- ¼ cup dry white wine
- Juice of 1 lemon
- 2 garlic cloves, minced
- ¼ teaspoon freshly ground black pepper

1. In a large skillet, heat 1½ teaspoons of oil over medium heat.
2. Add the asparagus and sauté for 5 to 6 minutes until just tender, stirring regularly. Remove from the skillet and cover with aluminum foil to keep warm.
3. Add the remaining 1½ teaspoons of oil and the butter to the skillet. When the butter is melted and sizzling, place the scallops in a single layer in the skillet. Cook for about 3 minutes on one side until nicely browned. Use tongs to gently loosen and flip the scallops, and cook on the other side for another 3 minutes until browned and cooked through. Remove and cover with foil to keep

warm.

4. In the same skillet, combine the wine, lemon juice, garlic, and pepper. Bring to a simmer for 1 to 2 minutes, stirring to mix in any browned pieces left in the pan.

5. Return the asparagus and the cooked scallops to the skillet to coat with the sauce. Serve warm.

*Per Serving:*calories: 252 / fat: 7g / protein: 26g / carbs: 15g / sugars: 3g / fiber: 2g / sodium: 493mg

Salmon en Papillote

Prep time: 15 minutes / Cook time: 15 minutes / Serves 2

- For the roasted vegetables
- ½ pound fresh green beans, trimmed
- ½ onion, cut into ¼-inch-thick slices
- 1 tablespoon extra-virgin olive oil
- 1 teaspoon capers (optional)
- For the salmon
- 2 teaspoons extra-virgin olive oil, divided
- 2 medium parsnips, cut into ¼-inch-thick rounds, divided
- 2 (4-ounce) salmon fillets
- 2 garlic cloves, thinly sliced, divided
- 1 lemon, divided (½ cut into slices, the other ½ cut into 2 wedges)
- 1 tablespoon chopped fresh thyme, divided
- Kosher salt
- Freshly ground black pepper

To make the roasted vegetables: 1. Preheat the oven to 400°F. Line a baking sheet with parchment paper.

2. In a medium bowl, toss the green beans, onion, extra-virgin olive oil, and capers (if using) until well coated.

3. Spread the vegetables on half of the baking sheet and set aside until the salmon is ready to bake. To make the salmon: 4. Cut two pieces of parchment paper, fold them in half, and cut each into a heart shape (about 10 to 12 inches in circumference). Lightly brush the parchment with ½ teaspoon of extra-virgin olive oil.

5. Open one of the hearts and place half the parsnips on the right half in the center, fanning them out. Place one piece of salmon on the fanned parsnips. Add half the garlic, half the lemon slices, half the thyme, ½ teaspoon of extra-virgin olive oil, and a pinch each of kosher salt and pepper.

6. Seal the packet by folding the left half of the heart over the right side. Fold along the edge of the heart and create a seal. Repeat with the other piece of parchment.

7. Place the packets on the empty side of the baking sheet and bake until the salmon is cooked through, 10 to 15 minutes. Allow the fish to rest a few

minutes before serving with the roasted green beans and remaining lemon wedges.

8. Store any leftovers in an airtight container in the refrigerator for 1 to 2 days.

*Per Serving:*calories: 389 / fat: 17g / protein: 28g / carbs: 35g / sugars: 11g / fiber: 10g / sodium: 261mg

Shrimp Stir-Fry

Prep time: 5 minutes / Cook time: 15 minutes / Serves 4

- For The Sauce
- ½ cup water
- 2½ tablespoons low-sodium soy sauce
- 2 tablespoons honey
- 1 tablespoon rice vinegar
- ¼ teaspoon garlic powder
- Pinch ground ginger
- 1 tablespoon cornstarch
- For The Stir-Fry
- 8 cups frozen vegetable stir-fry mix
- 2 tablespoons sesame oil
- 40 medium fresh shrimp, peeled and deveined

Make The Sauce: 1. In a small saucepan, whisk together the water, soy sauce, honey, rice vinegar, garlic powder, and ginger. Add the cornstarch and whisk until fully incorporated.

2. Bring the sauce to a boil over medium heat. Boil for 1 minute to thicken. Remove the sauce from the heat and set aside.

Make The Stir-Fry: 1. Heat a large saucepan over medium-high heat. When hot, put the vegetable stir-fry mix into the pan, and cook for 7 to 10 minutes, stirring occasionally until the water completely evaporates.

2. Reduce the heat to medium-low, add the oil and shrimp, and stir. Cook for about 3 minutes, or until the shrimp are pink and opaque.

3. Add the sauce to the shrimp and vegetables and stir to coat. Cook for 2 minutes more.

*Per Serving:*calories: 297 / fat: 17g / protein: 24g / carbs: 14g / sugars: 9g / fiber: 2g / sodium: 454mg

Grilled Scallop Kabobs

Prep time: 15 minutes / Cook time: 20 minutes / Serves 6

- 15 ounces pineapple chunks, packed in their own juice, undrained
- ¼ cup dry white wine
- ¼ cup light soy sauce
- 2 tablespoons minced fresh parsley
- 4 garlic cloves, minced
- ⅛ teaspoon freshly ground black pepper
- 1 pound scallops
- 18 large cherry tomatoes
- 1 large green bell pepper, cut into 1-inch squares

- 18 medium mushroom caps

1. Drain the pineapple, reserving the juice. In a shallow baking dish, combine the pineapple juice, wine, soy sauce, parsley, garlic, and pepper. Mix well.
2. Add the pineapple, scallops, tomatoes, green pepper, and mushrooms to the marinade. Marinate 30 minutes at room temperature, stirring occasionally.
3. Alternate pineapple, scallops, and vegetables on metal or wooden skewers (remember to soak wooden skewers in water before using).
4. Grill the kabobs over medium-hot coals about 4 to 5 inches from the heat, turning frequently, for 5 to 7 minutes.

Per Serving: *calories: 132 / fat: 1g / protein: 13g / carbs: 18g / sugars: 10g / fiber: 3g / sodium: 587mg*

Apple Cider Mussels

Prep time: 10 minutes / Cook time: 2 minutes / Serves 5

- 2 pounds (907 g) mussels, cleaned, peeled
- 1 teaspoon onion powder
- 1 teaspoon ground cumin
- 1 tablespoon avocado oil
- ¼ cup apple cider vinegar

1. Mix mussels with onion powder, ground cumin, avocado oil, and apple cider vinegar.
2. Put the mussels in the air fryer and cook at 395°F (202°C) for 2 minutes.

Per Serving: *calorie: 200 / fat: 6g / protein: 24g / carbs: 8g / sugars: 0g / fiber: 1g / sodium: 300mg*

Avo-Tuna with Croutons

Prep time: 10 minutes / Cook time: 0 minutes / Serves 3

- 2 (5-ounce) cans chunk-light tuna, drained
- 2 tablespoons low-fat mayonnaise
- ½ teaspoon freshly ground black pepper
- 3 avocados, halved and pitted
- 6 tablespoons packaged croutons

1. In a medium bowl, combine the tuna, mayonnaise, and pepper, and mix well.
2. Top the avocados with the tuna mixture and croutons.

Per Serving: *calories: 441 / fat: 32g / protein: 23g / carbs: 22g / sugars: 2g / fiber: 14g / sodium: 284mg*

Salade Niçoise with Oil-Packed Tuna

Prep time: 5 minutes / Cook time: 20 minutes / Serves 4

- 8 ounces small red potatoes, quartered
- 8 ounces green beans, trimmed
- 4 large eggs

- french vinaigrette
- 2 tablespoons extra-virgin olive oil
- 2 tablespoons cold-pressed avocado oil
- 2 tablespoons white wine vinegar
- 1 tablespoon water
- 1 teaspoon Dijon mustard
- ½ teaspoon dried oregano
- ¼ teaspoon fine sea salt
- 1 tablespoon minced shallot
- 2 hearts romaine lettuce, leaves separated and torn into bite-size pieces
- ½ cup grape tomatoes, halved
- ¼ cup pitted Niçoise or Greek olives
- One 7 ounces can oil-packed tuna, drained and flaked
- Freshly ground black pepper
- 1 tablespoon chopped fresh flat-leaf parsley

1. Pour 1 cup water into the Instant Pot and place a steamer basket into the pot. Add the potatoes, green beans, and eggs to the basket.
2. Secure the lid and set the Pressure Release to Sealing. Select the Steam setting and set the cooking time for 3 minutes at high pressure. (The pot will take about 15 minutes to come up to pressure before the cooking program begins.)
3. To make the vinaigrette: While the vegetables and eggs are steaming, in a small jar or other small container with a tight-fitting lid, combine the olive oil, avocado oil, vinegar, water, mustard, oregano, salt, and shallot and shake vigorously to emulsify. Set aside.
4. Prepare an ice bath.
5. When the cooking program ends, perform a quick release by moving the Pressure Release to Venting. Open the pot and, wearing heat-resistant mitts, lift out the steamer basket. Using tongs, transfer the eggs and green beans to the ice bath, leaving the potatoes in the steamer basket.
6. While the eggs and green beans are cooling, divide the lettuce, tomatoes, olives, and tuna among four shallow individual bowls. Drain the eggs and green beans. Peel and halve the eggs lengthwise, then arrange them on the salads along with the green beans and potatoes.
7. Spoon the vinaigrette over the salads and sprinkle with the pepper and parsley. Serve right away.

Per Serving: *calories: 367 / fat: 23g / protein: 20g / carbs: 23g / sugars: 7g / fiber: 4g / sodium: 268mg*

Peppercorn-Crusted Baked Salmon

Prep time: 5 minutes / Cook time: 20 minutes / Serves 4

- Nonstick cooking spray
- ½ teaspoon freshly ground black pepper
- ¼ teaspoon salt

- Zest and juice of ½ lemon
- ¼ teaspoon dried thyme
- 1 pound salmon fillet

1. Preheat the oven to 425°F. Spray a baking sheet with nonstick cooking spray.
2. In a small bowl, combine the pepper, salt, lemon zest and juice, and thyme. Stir to combine.
3. Place the salmon on the prepared baking sheet, skin-side down. Spread the seasoning mixture evenly over the fillet.
4. Bake for 15 to 20 minutes, depending on the thickness of the fillet, until the flesh flakes easily.

Per Serving:calories: 163 / fat: 7g / protein: 23g / carbs: 1g / sugars: 0g / fiber: 0g / sodium: 167mg

Lemony Salmon

Prep time: 30 minutes / Cook time: 10 minutes / Serves 4

- 1½ pounds (680 g) salmon steak
- ½ teaspoon grated lemon zest
- Freshly cracked mixed peppercorns, to taste
- ⅓ cup lemon juice
- Fresh chopped chives, for garnish
- ½ cup dry white wine
- ½ teaspoon fresh cilantro, chopped
- Fine sea salt, to taste

1. To prepare the marinade, place all ingredients, except for salmon steak and chives, in a deep pan. Bring to a boil over medium-high flame until it has reduced by half. Allow it to cool down.
2. After that, allow salmon steak to marinate in the refrigerator approximately 40 minutes. Discard the marinade and transfer the fish steak to the preheated air fryer.
3. Air fry at 400ºF (204ºC) for 9 to 10 minutes. To finish, brush hot fish steaks with the reserved marinade, garnish with fresh chopped chives, and serve right away!

Per Serving:calorie: 300 / fat: 20g / protein: 20g / carbs: 10g / sugars: 2g / fiber: 6g / sodium: 400mg

Herb-Crusted Halibut

Prep time: 10 minutes / Cook time: 20 minutes / Serves 4

- 4 (5-ounce) halibut fillets
- Extra-virgin olive oil, for brushing
- ½ cup coarsely ground unsalted pistachios
- 1 tablespoon chopped fresh parsley
- 1 teaspoon chopped fresh thyme
- 1 teaspoon chopped fresh basil
- Pinch sea salt
- Pinch freshly ground black pepper

1. Preheat the oven to 350°F.
2. Line a baking sheet with parchment paper.

3. Pat the halibut fillets dry with a paper towel and place them on the baking sheet.
4. Brush the halibut generously with olive oil.
5. In a small bowl, stir together the pistachios, parsley, thyme, basil, salt, and pepper.
6. Spoon the nut and herb mixture evenly on the fish, spreading it out so the tops of the fillets are covered.
7. Bake the halibut until it flakes when pressed with a fork, about 20 minutes.
8. Serve immediately.

Per Serving:calories: 351 / fat: 27g / protein: 24g / carbs: 4g / sugars: 1g / fiber: 2g / sodium: 214mg

Baked Garlic Scampi

Prep time: 5 minutes / Cook time: 10 minutes / Serves 4

- 1 tablespoon extra-virgin olive oil
- ¼ teaspoon salt
- 7 garlic cloves, crushed
- 2 tablespoons chopped fresh parsley, divided
- 1 pound large shrimp, shelled (with tails left on) and deveined
- Juice and zest of 1 lemon
- 2 cups baby arugula

1. Preheat the oven to 350 degrees. Grease a 13-x-9-x-2-inch baking pan with the olive oil. Add the salt, garlic, and 1 tablespoon of the parsley in a medium bowl; mix well, and set aside.
2. Arrange the shrimp in a single layer in the baking pan, and bake for 3 minutes, uncovered. Turn the shrimp, and sprinkle with the lemon peel, lemon juice, and the remaining 1 tablespoon of parsley. Continue to bake 1–2 minutes more until the shrimp are bright pink and tender.
3. Remove the shrimp from the oven. Place the arugula on a serving platter, and top with the shrimp. Spoon the garlic mixture over the shrimp and arugula, and serve.

Per Serving:calories: 140 / fat: 4g / protein: 23g / carbs: 3g / sugars: 1g / fiber: 0g / sodium: 285mg

Shrimp Burgers with Fruity Salsa and Salad

Prep time: 15 minutes / Cook time: 10 minutes / Serves 4

- For The Salsa:
- 1 cup diced mango
- 1 avocado, diced
- 1 scallion, both white and green parts, finely chopped
- 1 tablespoon chopped fresh cilantro
- Juice of 1 lime
- ¼ teaspoon freshly ground black pepper
- For The Burgers:
- 1 pound shrimp, peeled and deveined

- 1 large egg
- ½ red bell pepper, seeded and coarsely chopped
- ¼ cup chopped scallions, both white and green parts
- 2 tablespoons fresh chopped cilantro
- 2 garlic cloves
- ¼ teaspoon freshly ground black pepper
- 1 tablespoon extra-virgin olive oil
- 4 cups mixed salad greens

Make The Salsa: In a small bowl, toss the mango, avocado, scallion, and cilantro. Sprinkle with the lime juice and pepper. Mix gently to combine and set aside. Make The Burgers: 1. In the bowl of a food processor, add half the shrimp and process until coarsely puréed. Add the egg, bell pepper, scallions, cilantro, and garlic, and process until uniformly chopped. Transfer to a large mixing bowl.

2. Using a sharp knife, chop the remaining half pound of shrimp into small pieces. Add to the puréed mixture and stir well to combine. Add the pepper and stir well. Form the mixture into 4 patties of equal size. Arrange on a plate, cover, and refrigerate for 30 minutes.
3. In a large skillet, heat the olive oil over medium heat. Cook the burgers for 3 minutes on each side until browned and cooked through.
4. On each of 4 plates, arrange 1 cup of salad greens, and top with a scoop of salsa and a shrimp burger.

Per Serving:*calories: 229 / fat: 11g / protein: 19g / carbs: 14g / sugars: 7g / fiber: 4g / sodium: 200mg*

Shrimp Étouffée

Prep time: 20 minutes / Cook time: 30 minutes / Serves 4 to 6

- 2 cups store-bought low-sodium vegetable broth, divided
- ¼ cup whole-wheat flour
- 1 small onion, finely chopped
- 2 celery stalks including leaves, finely chopped
- 1 medium green bell pepper, finely chopped
- 1 medium poblano pepper, finely chopped
- 3 garlic cloves, minced
- 1 tablespoon Creole seasoning
- 2 pounds medium shrimp, shelled and deveined
- ⅓ cup finely chopped chives, for garnish

1. In a Dutch oven, bring ½ cup of broth to a simmer over medium heat.
2. Stir in the flour and reduce the heat to low. Cook, stirring often, for 5 minutes, or until a thick paste is formed.
3. Add ½ cup of broth, the onion, celery, bell pepper, poblano pepper, and garlic and cook for 2 to 5 minutes, or until the vegetables have softened.

4. Slowly add the seasoning and remaining 1 cup of broth, ¼ cup at a time.
5. Add the shrimp and cook for about 5 minutes, or until just opaque.
6. Serve with the vegetable of your choice. Garnish with the chives.

Per Serving:*calories: 164 / fat: 1g / protein: 32g / carbs: 8g / sugars: 2g / fiber: 1g / sodium: 500mg*

Lemon Pepper Salmon

Prep time: 5 minutes / Cook time: 20 minutes / Serves 4

- Avocado oil cooking spray
- 20 Brussels sprouts, halved lengthwise
- 4 (4-ounce) skinless salmon fillets
- ½ teaspoon garlic powder
- ½ teaspoon freshly ground black pepper
- ¼ teaspoon salt
- 2 teaspoons freshly squeezed lemon juice

1. Heat a large skillet over medium-low heat. When hot, coat the cooking surface with cooking spray, and put the Brussels sprouts cut-side down in the skillet. Cover and cook for 5 minutes.
2. Meanwhile, season both sides of the salmon with the garlic powder, pepper, and salt.
3. Flip the Brussels sprouts, and move them to one side of the skillet. Add the salmon and cook, uncovered, for 4 to 6 minutes.
4. Check the Brussels sprouts. When they are tender, remove them from the skillet and set them aside.
5. Flip the salmon fillets. Cook for 4 to 6 more minutes, or until the salmon is opaque and flakes easily with a fork. Remove the salmon from the skillet, and let it rest for 5 minutes.
6. Divide the Brussels sprouts into four equal portions and add 1 salmon fillet to each portion. Sprinkle the lemon juice on top and serve.

Per Serving:*calories: 163 / fat: 7g / protein: 23g / carbs: 1g / sugars: 0g / fiber: 0g / sodium: 167mg*

Friday Night Fish Fry

Prep time: 10 minutes / Cook time: 10 minutes / Serves 4

- 1 large egg
- ½ cup powdered Parmesan cheese (about 1½ ounces / 43 g)
- 1 teaspoon smoked paprika
- ¼ teaspoon celery salt
- ¼ teaspoon ground black pepper
- 4 (4-ounce / 113-g) cod fillets
- Chopped fresh oregano or parsley, for garnish (optional)
- Lemon slices, for serving (optional)

1. Spray the air fryer basket with avocado oil. Preheat the air fryer to 400ºF (204ºC).

2. Crack the egg in a shallow bowl and beat it lightly with a fork. Combine the Parmesan cheese, paprika, celery salt, and pepper in a separate shallow bowl.
3. One at a time, dip the fillets into the egg, then dredge them in the Parmesan mixture. Using your hands, press the Parmesan onto the fillets to form a nice crust. As you finish, place the fish in the air fryer basket.
4. Air fry the fish in the air fryer for 10 minutes, or until it is cooked through and flakes easily with a fork. Garnish with fresh oregano or parsley and serve with lemon slices, if desired.
5. Store leftovers in an airtight container in the refrigerator for up to 3 days. Reheat in a preheated 400°F (204°C) air fryer for 5 minutes, or until warmed through.

Per Serving:calorie: 300 / fat: 12g / protein: 40g / carbs: 6g / sugars: 1g / fiber: 0g / sodium: 800mg

Cajun Salmon

Prep time: 5 minutes / Cook time: 7 minutes / Serves 2

- 2 (4 ounces / 113 g) salmon fillets, skin removed
- 2 tablespoons unsalted butter, melted
- ⅛ teaspoon ground cayenne pepper
- ½ teaspoon garlic powder
- 1 teaspoon paprika
- ¼ teaspoon ground black pepper

1. Brush each fillet with butter.
2. Combine remaining ingredients in a small bowl and then rub onto fish. Place fillets into the air fryer basket.
3. Adjust the temperature to 390°F (199°C) and air fry for 7 minutes.
4. When fully cooked, internal temperature will be 145°F (63°C). Serve immediately.

Per Serving:calorie: 323 / fat: 26g / protein: 20g / carbs: 2g / sugars: 0g / fiber: 1g / sodium: 200mg

Snapper with Shallot and Tomato

Prep time: 20 minutes / Cook time: 15 minutes / Serves 2

- 2 snapper fillets
- 1 shallot, peeled and sliced
- 2 garlic cloves, halved
- 1 bell pepper, sliced
- 1 small-sized serrano pepper, sliced
- 1 tomato, sliced
- 1 tablespoon olive oil
- ¼ teaspoon freshly ground black pepper
- ½ teaspoon paprika
- Sea salt, to taste
- 2 bay leaves

1. Place two parchment sheets on a working surface.

Place the fish in the center of one side of the parchment paper.
2. Top with the shallot, garlic, peppers, and tomato. Drizzle olive oil over the fish and vegetables. Season with black pepper, paprika, and salt. Add the bay leaves.
3. Fold over the other half of the parchment. Now, fold the paper around the edges tightly and create a half moon shape, sealing the fish inside.
4. Cook in the preheated air fryer at 390°F (199°C) for 15 minutes. Serve warm.

Per Serving:calories: 325 / fat: 10g / protein: 47g / carbs: 11g / sugars: 2g/fiber: 2g / sodium: 146mg

Scallops in Lemon-Butter Sauce

Prep time: 10 minutes / Cook time: 6 minutes / Serves 2

- 8 large dry sea scallops (about ¾ pound / 340 g)
- Salt and freshly ground black pepper, to taste
- 2 tablespoons olive oil
- 2 tablespoons unsalted butter, melted
- 2 tablespoons chopped flat-leaf parsley
- 1 tablespoon fresh lemon juice
- 2 teaspoons capers, drained and chopped
- 1 teaspoon grated lemon zest
- 1 clove garlic, minced

1. Preheat the air fryer to 400°F (204°C).
2. Use a paper towel to pat the scallops dry. Sprinkle lightly with salt and pepper. Brush with the olive oil. Arrange the scallops in a single layer in the air fryer basket. Pausing halfway through the cooking time to turn the scallops, air fry for about 6 minutes until firm and opaque.
3. Meanwhile, in a small bowl, combine the oil, butter, parsley, lemon juice, capers, lemon zest, and garlic. Drizzle over the scallops just before serving.

Per Serving:calorie: 350 / fat: 22g / protein: 30g / carbs: 4g / sugars: 1g / fiber: 1g / sodium: 400mg

Marinated Swordfish Skewers

Prep time: 30 minutes / Cook time: 6 to 8 minutes / Serves 4

- 1 pound (454 g) filleted swordfish
- ¼ cup avocado oil
- 2 tablespoons freshly squeezed lemon juice
- 1 tablespoon minced fresh parsley
- 2 teaspoons Dijon mustard
- Sea salt and freshly ground black pepper, to taste
- 3 ounces (85 g) cherry tomatoes

1. Cut the fish into 1½-inch chunks, picking out any remaining bones.
2. In a large bowl, whisk together the oil, lemon juice, parsley, and Dijon mustard. Season to taste

with salt and pepper. Add the fish and toss to coat the pieces. Cover and marinate the fish chunks in the refrigerator for 30 minutes.
3. Remove the fish from the marinade. Thread the fish and cherry tomatoes on 4 skewers, alternating as you go.
4. Set the air fryer to 400°F (204°C). Place the skewers in the air fryer basket and air fry for 3 minutes. Flip the skewers and cook for 3 to 5 minutes longer, until the fish is cooked through and an instant-read thermometer reads 140°F (60°C).

Per Serving:calories: 291 / fat: 21g / protein: 23g / carbs: 2g / sugars: 1g / fiber: 0g / sodium: 121mg

Almond Catfish

Prep time: 10 minutes / Cook time: 12 minutes / Serves 4

• 2 pounds (907 g) catfish fillet
• ½ cup almond flour
• 2 eggs, beaten
• 1 teaspoon salt
• 1 teaspoon avocado oil

1. Sprinkle the catfish fillet with salt and dip in the eggs.
2. Then coat the fish in the almond flour and put in the air fryer basket. Sprinkle the fish with avocado oil.
3. Cook the fish for 6 minutes per side at 380°F (193°C).

Per Serving:calories: 308 / fat: 10g / protein: 42g / carbs: 11g / sugars: 0g / fiber: 2g / sodium: 610mg

Rainbow Salmon Kebabs

Prep time: 10 minutes / Cook time: 8 minutes / Serves 2

• 6 ounces (170 g) boneless, skinless salmon, cut into 1-inch cubes
• ¼ medium red onion, peeled and cut into 1-inch pieces
• ½ medium yellow bell pepper, seeded and cut into 1-inch pieces
• ½ medium zucchini, trimmed and cut into ½-inch slices
• 1 tablespoon olive oil
• ½ teaspoon salt
• ¼ teaspoon ground black pepper

1. Using one (6-inch) skewer, skewer 1 piece salmon, then 1 piece onion, 1 piece bell pepper, and finally 1 piece zucchini. Repeat this pattern with additional skewers to make four kebabs total. Drizzle with olive oil and sprinkle with salt and black pepper.
2. Place kebabs into ungreased air fryer basket. Adjust the temperature to 400°F (204°C) and air

fry for 8 minutes, turning kebabs halfway through cooking. Salmon will easily flake and have an internal temperature of at least 145°F (63°C) when done; vegetables will be tender. Serve warm.

Per Serving:calorie: 300 / fat: 18g / protein: 26g / carbs: 10g / sugars: 4g / fiber: 3g / sodium: 600mg

Sea Bass with Ginger Sauce

Prep time: 5 minutes / Cook time: 15 minutes / Serves 2

• Two 4-ounce sea bass filets
• 1 tablespoon extra-virgin olive oil
• 2 tablespoons minced fresh ginger
• 2 garlic cloves, minced
• ⅓ cup minced scallions
• 4 teaspoons chopped cilantro
• 1 tablespoon light soy sauce

1. In a medium steamer, add water and bring to a boil. Arrange the filets on the steamer rack. Cover, and steam for 6–8 minutes.
2. Meanwhile, in a small skillet, heat the oil over medium-high heat. Add the ginger and garlic, and sauté for 2–3 minutes.
3. Transfer the steamed filets to a platter. Pour the ginger oil over the filets, and top with scallions, cilantro, and soy sauce.

Per Serving:calories: 207 / fat: 11g / protein: 22g / carbs: 5g / sugars: 2g / fiber: 1g / sodium: 202mg

Catfish with Corn and Pepper Relish

Prep time: 10 minutes / Cook time: 10 minutes / Serves 4

• 3 tablespoons extra-virgin olive oil, divided
• 4 (5-ounce) catfish fillets
• ¼ teaspoon salt
• ¼ teaspoon freshly ground black pepper
• 1 (15-ounce) can low-sodium black beans, drained and rinsed
• 1 cup frozen corn
• 1 medium red bell pepper, diced
• 1 tablespoon apple cider vinegar
• 3 tablespoons chopped scallions

1. Use 1½ tablespoons of oil to coat both sides of the catfish fillets, then season the fillets with the salt and pepper.
2. Heat a small saucepan over medium-high heat. Put the remaining 1½ tablespoons of oil, beans, corn, bell pepper, and vinegar in the pan and stir. Cover and cook for 5 minutes.
3. Place the catfish fillets on top of the relish mixture and cover. Cook for 5 to 7 minutes.
4. Serve each catfish fillet with one-quarter of the relish and top with the scallions.

Per Serving:calories: 379 / fat: 15g / protein: 32g / carbs:

31g / sugars: 2g / fiber: 10g / sodium: 366mg

Spicy Corn and Shrimp Salad in Avocado

Prep time: 10 minutes / Cook time: 0 minutes / Serves 2

- ¼ cup mayonnaise
- 1 teaspoon sriracha (or to taste)
- ½ teaspoon lemon zest
- ¼ teaspoon sea salt
- 4 ounces cooked baby shrimp
- ½ cup cooked and cooled corn kernels
- ½ red bell pepper, seeded and chopped
- 1 avocado, halved lengthwise

1. In a medium bowl, combine the mayonnaise, sriracha, lemon zest, and salt.
2. Add the shrimp, corn, and bell pepper. Mix to combine.
3. Spoon the mixture into the avocado halves.

Per Serving:*calories: 354 / fat: 25g / protein: 17g / carbs: 21g / sugars: 2g / fiber: 9g / sodium: 600mg*

Blackened Pollock

Prep time: 15 minutes / Cook time: 10 minutes / Serves 2

- 8 ounces pollock (or other white fish) fillet, skinned and halved
- 3 teaspoons extra-virgin olive oil, divided
- 1 teaspoon blackening seasoning, or Cajun seasoning, divided
- ¼ cup thinly sliced onion
- 4 cups baby spinach, divided
- ½ small grapefruit, peeled and segmented
- 2 tablespoons shaved fennel
- 2 tablespoons pepitas
- ½ small avocado, peeled, pitted, and sliced, divided

1. Brush both sides of each pollock half with 1½ teaspoons of olive oil.
2. Rub each half all over with ½ teaspoon of blackening seasoning.
3. In a large heavy skillet set over high heat, cook the pollock and onions for 2 to 3 minutes, until blackened. Turn the fillets. Cook for 2 to 3 minutes more, or until blackened and the fish flakes easily with a fork.
4. Put 2 cups of arugula on each serving plate. Top each with 1 pollock half.

5. Top each serving with half of the grapefruit, fennel, pepitas, and avocado.

Per Serving:*calories: 302 / fat: 19g / protein: 20g / carbs: 16g / sugars: 5g / fiber: 8g / sodium: 436mg*

Spicy Shrimp Fajitas

Prep time: 30 minutes / Cook time: 20 minutes / Makes 6 fajitas

- arinade
- 1 tablespoon lime juice
- 1 tablespoon olive or canola oil
- ¼ teaspoon salt
- 1 teaspoon chili powder
- 1 teaspoon ground cumin
- 2 cloves garlic, crushed
- Pinch ground red pepper (cayenne)
- Fajitas
- 2 pounds uncooked deveined peeled medium shrimp, thawed if frozen, tail shells removed
- 2 medium red bell peppers, cut into strips (2 cups)
- 1 medium red onion, sliced (2 cups)
- Olive oil cooking spray
- 6 flour tortillas (8 inch)
- ¾ cup refrigerated guacamole (from 14-ounces package)

1. Heat gas or charcoal grill. In 1-gallon resealable food-storage plastic bag, mix marinade ingredients. Add shrimp; seal bag and toss to coat. Set aside while grilling vegetables, turning bag once.
2. In medium bowl, place bell peppers and onion; spray with cooking spray. Place vegetables in grill basket (grill "wok"). Wrap tortillas in foil; set aside.
3. Place basket on grill rack over medium heat. Cover grill; cook 10 minutes, turning vegetables once.
4. Drain shrimp; discard marinade. Add shrimp to grill basket. Cover grill; cook 5 to 7 minutes longer, turning shrimp and vegetables once, until shrimp are pink. Place wrapped tortillas on grill. Cook 2 minutes, turning once, until warm.
5. On each tortilla, place shrimp, vegetables and guacamole; fold tortilla over filling.

Per Serving:*calories: 310 / fat: 10g / protein:27g / carbs: 29g / sugars: 4g / fiber: 2g / sodium: 770mg*

Chapter 6 Snacks and Appetizers

Crab-Filled Mushrooms

Prep time: 5 minutes / Cook time: 25 minutes / Serves 10

- 20 large fresh mushroom caps
- 6 ounces canned crabmeat, rinsed, drained, and flaked
- ½ cup crushed whole-wheat crackers
- 2 tablespoons chopped fresh parsley
- 2 tablespoons finely chopped green onion
- ⅛ teaspoon freshly ground black pepper
- ¼ cup chopped pimiento
- 3 tablespoons extra-virgin olive oil
- 10 tablespoons wheat germ

1. Preheat the oven to 350 degrees. Clean the mushrooms by dusting off any dirt on the cap with a mushroom brush or paper towel; remove the stems.
2. In a small mixing bowl, combine the crabmeat, crackers, parsley, onion, and pepper.
3. Place the mushroom caps in a 13-x-9-x-2-inch baking dish, crown side down. Stuff some of the crabmeat filling into each cap. Place a little pimiento on top of the filling.
4. Drizzle the olive oil over the caps and sprinkle each cap with ½ tablespoon wheat germ. Bake for 15–17 minutes. Transfer to a serving platter, and serve hot.

Per Serving:calorie: 113 / fat: 6g / protein: 7g / carbs: 9g / sugars: 1g / fiber: 2g / sodium: 77mg

Fresh Dill Dip

Prep time: 5 minutes / Cook time: 5 minutes / Serves 6

- 1 cup plain fat-free yogurt
- ¼ teaspoon salt
- ¼ teaspoon freshly ground black pepper
- ¼ cup minced parsley
- 2 tablespoons finely chopped fresh chives
- 1 tablespoon finely chopped fresh dill
- 1 tablespoon apple cider vinegar

1. In a small bowl, combine all the ingredients. Chill for 2 to 4 hours. Serve with fresh cut vegetables.

Per Serving:calorie: 20 / fat: 0g / protein: 2g / carbs: 3g / sugars: 2g / fiber: 0g / sodium: 120mg

Smoky Spinach Hummus with Popcorn Chips

Prep time: 10 minutes / Cook time: 0 minutes / Serves 12

- 1 can (15 ounces) chickpeas (garbanzo beans), drained, liquid reserved
- 1 cup chopped fresh spinach leaves
- 2 tablespoons lemon juice
- 2 tablespoons sesame tahini paste (from 16 ounces. jar)
- 2 teaspoons smoked Spanish paprika
- 1 teaspoon ground cumin
- ½ teaspoon salt
- 2 tablespoons chopped red bell pepper, if desired
- 6 ounces popcorn snack chips

1. In food processor, place chickpeas, ¼ cup of the reserved liquid, spinach, lemon juice, tahini paste, paprika, cumin and salt. Cover; process 30 seconds, using quick on-and-off motions; scrape side.
2. Add additional reserved bean liquid, 1 tablespoon at a time, covering and processing, using quick on-and-off motions, until smooth and desired dipping consistency. Garnish with bell pepper. Serve with popcorn snack chips.

Per Serving:calories: 140 / fat: 4g / protein: 4g / carbs: 22g / sugars: 0g / fiber: 3g / sodium: 270mg

Cocoa Coated Almonds

Prep time: 5 minutes / Cook time: 15 minutes / Serves 4

- 1 cup almonds
- 1 tablespoon cocoa powder
- 2 packets powdered stevia

1. Preheat the oven to 350°F. Line a baking sheet with parchment paper.
2. Spread the almonds in a single layer on the baking sheet. Bake for 5 minutes.
3. While the almonds bake, in a small bowl, mix the cocoa and stevia well. Add the hot almonds to the bowl. Toss to combine.
4. Return the almonds to the baking sheet and bake until fragrant, about 5 minutes more.

Per Serving:calorie: 143 / fat: 12g / protein: 5g / carbs: 6g / sugars: 1g / fiber: 3g / sodium: 1mg

Guacamole with Jicama

Prep time: 5 minutes / Cook time: 0 minutes / Serves 4

- 1 avocado, cut into cubes
- Juice of ½ lime
- 2 tablespoons finely chopped red onion
- 2 tablespoons chopped fresh cilantro
- 1 garlic clove, minced
- ¼ teaspoon sea salt
- 1 cup sliced jicama

1. In a small bowl, combine the avocado, lime juice, onion, cilantro, garlic, and salt. Mash lightly with a fork.
2. Serve with the jicama for dipping.

Creamy Spinach Dip

Prep time: 13 minutes / Cook time: 5 minutes / Serves 11

- 8 ounces low-fat cream cheese
- 1 cup low-fat sour cream
- ½ cup finely chopped onion
- ½ cup no-sodium vegetable broth
- 5 cloves garlic, minced
- ½ teaspoon salt
- ¼ teaspoon black pepper
- 10 ounces frozen spinach
- 12 ounces reduced-fat shredded Monterey Jack cheese
- 12 ounces reduced-fat shredded Parmesan cheese

1. Add cream cheese, sour cream, onion, vegetable broth, garlic, salt, pepper, and spinach to the inner pot of the Instant Pot.
2. Secure lid, make sure vent is set to sealing, and set to the Bean/Chili setting on high pressure for 5 minutes.
3. When done, do a manual release.
4. Add the cheeses and mix well until creamy and well combined.

*Per Serving:*calorie: 274 / fat: 18g / protein: 19g / carbs: 10g / sugars: 3g / fiber: 1g / sodium: 948mg

Low-Sugar Blueberry Muffins

Prep time: 5 minutes / Cook time: 20 to 25 minutes / Makes 12 muffins

- 2 large eggs
- 1½ cups (144 g) almond flour
- 1 cup (80 g) gluten-free rolled oats
- ½ cup (120 ml) pure maple syrup
- ½ cup (120 ml) avocado oil
- 1 teaspoon baking powder
- 1 teaspoon ground cinnamon
- ½ teaspoon pure vanilla extract
- ½ teaspoon pure almond extract
- 1 cup (150 g) fresh or frozen blueberries

1. Preheat the oven to 350°F (177°C). Line a 12-well muffin pan with paper liners or spray the wells with cooking oil spray.
2. In a blender, combine the eggs, almond flour, oats, maple syrup, oil, baking powder, cinnamon, vanilla, and almond extract. Blend the ingredients on high for 20 to 30 seconds, until the mixture is homogeneous.
3. Transfer the batter to a large bowl and gently stir in the blueberries.
4. Divide the batter evenly among the muffin wells. Bake the muffins for 20 to 25 minutes, until a toothpick inserted in the middle comes out clean.

5. Let the muffins rest for 5 minutes, then transfer them to a cooling rack.

*Per Serving:*calorie: 240 / fat: 18g / protein: 5g / carbs: 19g / sugars: 10g / fiber: 3g / sodium: 19mg

Green Goddess White Bean Dip

Prep time: 1 minutes / Cook time: 45 minutes / Makes 3 cups

- 1 cup dried navy, great Northern, or cannellini beans
- 4 cups water
- 2 teaspoons fine sea salt
- 3 tablespoons fresh lemon juice
- ¼ cup extra-virgin olive oil, plus 1 tablespoon
- ¼ cup firmly packed fresh flat-leaf parsley leaves
- 1 bunch chives, chopped
- Leaves from 2 tarragon sprigs
- Freshly ground black pepper

1. Combine the beans, water, and 1 teaspoon of the salt in the Instant Pot and stir to dissolve the salt.
2. Secure the lid and set the Pressure Release to Sealing. Select the Bean/Chili, Pressure Cook, or Manual setting and set the cooking time for 30 minutes at high pressure if using navy or Great Northern beans or 40 minutes at high pressure if using cannellini beans. (The pot will take about 15 minutes to come up to pressure before the cooking program begins.)
3. When the cooking program ends, let the pressure release naturally for 15 minutes, then move the Pressure Release to Venting to release any remaining steam. Open the pot and scoop out and reserve ½ cup of the cooking liquid. Wearing heat-resistant mitts, lift out the inner pot and drain the beans in a colander.
4. In a food processor or blender, combine the beans, ½ cup cooking liquid, lemon juice, ¼ cup olive oil, ½ teaspoon parsley, chives, tarragon, remaining 1 teaspoon salt, and ½ teaspoon pepper. Process or blend on medium speed, stopping to scrape down the sides of the container as needed, for about 1 minute, until the mixture is smooth.
5. Transfer the dip to a serving bowl. Drizzle with the remaining 1 tablespoon olive oil and sprinkle with a few grinds of pepper. The dip will keep in an airtight container in the refrigerator for up to 1 week. Serve at room temperature or chilled.

*Per Serving:*calorie: 70 / fat: 5g / protein: 3g / carbs: 8g / sugars: 1g / fiber: 4g / sodium: 782mg

Blood Sugar–Friendly Nutty Trail Mix

Prep time: 5 minutes / Cook time: 0 minutes / Serves 4

- ¼ cup (31 g) raw shelled pistachios
- ¼ cup (30 g) raw pecans

- ¼ cup (43 g) raw almonds
- ¼ cup (38 g) raisins
- ¼ cup (45 g) dairy-free dark chocolate chips

1. In a medium bowl, combine the pistachios, pecans, almonds, raisins, and chocolate chips.
2. Divide the trail mix into four portions.

Per Serving:calorie: 234 / fat: 17g / protein: 5g / carbs: 21g / sugars: 15g / fiber: 4g / sodium: 6mg

Creamy Apple-Cinnamon Quesadilla

Prep time: 15 minutes / Cook time: 10 minutes / Serves 4

- 1 tablespoon granulated sugar
- ½ teaspoon ground cinnamon
- ¼ cup reduced-fat cream cheese (from 8 ounces container)
- 1 tablespoon packed brown sugar
- 2 whole wheat tortillas (8 inch)
- ½ small apple, cut into ¼-inch slices (½ cup)
- Cooking spray

1. In small bowl, mix granulated sugar and ¼ teaspoon of the cinnamon; set aside. In another small bowl, mix cream cheese, brown sugar and remaining ¼ teaspoon cinnamon with spoon.
2. Spread cream cheese mixture over tortillas. Place apple slices on cream cheese mixture on 1 tortilla. Top with remaining tortilla, cheese side down. Spray both sides of quesadilla with cooking spray; sprinkle with cinnamon-sugar mixture.
3. Heat 10-inch nonstick skillet over medium heat. Add quesadilla; cook 2 to 3 minutes or until bottom is brown and crisp. Turn quesadilla; cook 2 to 3 minutes longer or until bottom is brown and crisp.
4. Transfer quesadilla from skillet to cutting board; let stand 2 to 3 minutes. Cut into 8 wedges to serve.

Per Serving:calories: 110 / fat: 3g / protein: 3g / carbs: 19g / sugars: 9g / fiber: 2g / sodium: 170mg

Broiled Shrimp with Garlic

Prep time: 5 minutes / Cook time: 10 minutes / Serves 12

- 2 pounds large shrimp, unshelled
- ⅓ cup extra-virgin olive oil
- 1 tablespoon lemon juice
- ¼ cup chopped scallions
- 1 tablespoon chopped garlic
- 2 teaspoons freshly ground black pepper
- 1 large lemon, sliced
- 4 tablespoons chopped fresh parsley

1. Set the oven to broil. Shell the uncooked shrimp, but do not remove the tails. With a small knife, split the shrimp down the back, and remove the vein. Wash the shrimp with cool water, and pat dry with paper towels.

2. In a medium skillet, over medium heat, heat the olive oil. Add the lemon juice, scallions, garlic, and pepper. Heat the mixture for 3 minutes. Set aside.
3. In a baking dish, arrange the shrimp and pour the olive oil mixture over the shrimp. Broil the shrimp 4–5 inches from the heat for 2 minutes per side, just until the shrimp turns bright pink. Transfer the shrimp to a platter and garnish with lemon slices and parsley. Pour the juices from the pan over the shrimp.

Per Serving:calorie: 92 / fat: 3g / protein: 15g / carbs: 1g / sugars: 0g / fiber: 0g / sodium: 142mg

Ginger and Mint Dip with Fruit

Prep time: 20 minutes / Cook time: 0 minutes / Serves 6

- Dip
- 1¼ cups plain fat-free yogurt
- ¼ cup packed brown sugar
- 2 teaspoons chopped fresh mint leaves
- 2 teaspoons grated gingerroot
- ½ teaspoon grated lemon peel
- Fruit Skewers
- 12 bamboo skewers (6 inch)
- 1 cup fresh raspberries
- 2 cups melon cubes (cantaloupe and/or honeydew)

1. In small bowl, mix dip ingredients with whisk until smooth. Cover; refrigerate at least 15 minutes to blend flavors.
2. On each skewer, alternately thread 3 raspberries and 2 melon cubes. Serve with dip.

Per Serving:calories: 100 / fat: 0g / protein: 3g / carbs: 20g / sugars: 17g / fiber: 2g / sodium: 50mg

Roasted Carrot and Chickpea Dip

Prep time: 10 minutes / Cook time: 15 minutes / Makes 4 cups

- 4 medium carrots, quartered lengthwise
- ¼ cup plus 2 teaspoons extra-virgin olive oil, divided
- Pinch kosher salt
- Pinch freshly ground black pepper
- 1 (15-ounce) can chickpeas, drained and rinsed
- 1 garlic clove, minced
- 1 red chile (optional)
- Zest and juice of 1 lemon
- 2 tablespoons tahini
- 1 tablespoon harissa
- ½ teaspoon ground cumin
- ¼ teaspoon ground coriander
- Pomegranate arils (seeds) (optional)
- Cilantro, chopped (optional)

1. Preheat the oven to 425°F. Line a baking sheet with parchment paper.

2. In a medium bowl, toss the carrots with 2 teaspoons of extra-virgin olive oil, the salt, and the pepper. Spread them in a single layer on the prepared baking sheet and roast until tender, about 15 minutes. Turn the carrots over halfway through.

3. Meanwhile, place the chickpeas, garlic, chile, lemon zest and juice, tahini, harissa, cumin, and coriander in a food processor. Set aside. Add the carrots to the processor when they are cooked. Pulse until the mixture is coarse. Scrape the bowl down, then turn the processor back on while you drizzle the remaining ¼ cup of extra-virgin olive oil through the feed tube of the machine. Adjust the seasonings as desired. If it's too thick, add water to thin.

4. Top with pomegranate seeds and chopped cilantro (if using,) and Serve with cut vegetables.

5. Store any leftovers in an airtight container in the refrigerator for up to 4 days.

Per Serving:calorie: 141 / fat: 10g / protein: 3g / carbs: 12g / sugars: 3g / fiber: 3g / sodium: 93mg

Southern Boiled Peanuts

Prep time: 5 minutes / Cook time: 1 hour 20 minutes / Makes 8 cups

- 1 pound raw jumbo peanuts in the shell
- 3 tablespoons fine sea salt

1. Remove the inner pot from the Instant Pot and add the peanuts to it. Cover the peanuts with water and use your hands to agitate them, loosening any dirt. Drain the peanuts in a colander, rinse out the pot, and return the peanuts to it. Return the inner pot to the Instant Pot housing.

2. Add the salt and 9 cups water to the pot and stir to dissolve the salt. Select a salad plate just small enough to fit inside the pot and set it on top of the peanuts to weight them down, submerging them all in the water.

3. Secure the lid and set the Pressure Release to Sealing. Select the Steam setting and set the cooking time for 1 hour at low pressure. (The pot will take about 20 minutes to come up to pressure before the cooking program begins.)

4. When the cooking program ends, let the pressure release naturally (this will take about 1 hour). Open the pot and, wearing heat-resistant mitts, remove the inner pot from the housing. Let the peanuts cool to room temperature in the brine (this will take about 1½ hours).

5. Serve at room temperature or chilled. Transfer the peanuts with their brine to an airtight container and refrigerate for up to 1 week.

Per Serving:calories: 306 / fat: 17g / protein: 26g / carbs: 12g / sugars: 2g / fiber: 4g / sodium: 303mg

Cucumber Roll-Ups

Prep time: 5 minutes / Cook time: 0 minutes / Serves 2 to 4

- 2 (6-inch) gluten-free wraps
- 2 tablespoons cream cheese
- 1 medium cucumber, cut into long strips
- 2 tablespoons fresh mint

1. Place the wraps on your work surface and spread them evenly with the cream cheese. Top with the cucumber and mint.

2. Roll the wraps up from one side to the other, kind of like a burrito. Slice into 1-inch bites or keep whole.

3. Serve.

4. Store any leftovers in an airtight container in the refrigerator for 1 to 2 days.

Per Serving:calorie: 70 / fat: 1g / protein: 4g / carbs: 12g / sugars: 3g / fiber: 2g / sodium: 183mg

No-Bake Coconut and Cashew Energy Bars

Prep time: 5 minutes / Cook time: 0 minutes / Makes 12 energy bars

- 1 cup (110 g) raw cashews
- 1 cup (80 g) unsweetened shredded coconut
- ½ cup (120 g) unsweetened nut butter of choice
- 2 tablespoons (30 ml) pure maple syrup

1. Line an 8 x 8–inch (20 x 20–cm) baking pan with parchment paper.

2. In a large food processor, combine the cashews and coconut. Pulse them for 15 to 20 seconds to form a powder.

3. Add the nut butter and maple syrup and process until a doughy paste is formed, scraping down the sides if needed.

4. Spread the dough into the prepared baking pan. Cover the dough with another sheet of parchment paper and press it flat.

5. Freeze the dough for 1 hour. Cut the dough into bars.

Per Serving:calorie: 169 / fat: 14g / protein: 4g / carbs: 10g / sugars: 3g / fiber: 2g / sodium: 6mg

Porcupine Meatballs

Prep time: 20 minutes / Cook time: 15 minutes / Serves 8

- 1 pound ground sirloin or turkey
- ½ cup raw brown rice, parboiled
- 1 egg
- ¼ cup finely minced onion
- 1 or 2 cloves garlic, minced
- ¼ teaspoon dried basil and/or oregano, optional
- 10¾-ounce can reduced-fat condensed tomato soup
- ½ soup can of water

1. Mix all ingredients, except tomato soup and water, in a bowl to combine well.

2. Form into balls about 1½-inch in diameter.
3. Mix tomato soup and water in the inner pot of the Instant Pot, then add the meatballs.
4. Secure the lid and make sure the vent is turned to sealing.
5. Press the Meat button and set for 15 minutes on high pressure.
6. Allow the pressure to release naturally after cook time is up.

Per Serving:calories: 141 / fat: 2g / protein: 16g / carbs: 14g / sugars: 3g / fiber: 1g / sodium: 176mg

Hummus

Prep time: 5 minutes / Cook time: 5 minutes / Serves 12

- One 15-ounce can chickpeas, drained (reserve a little liquid)
- 3 cloves garlic
- Juice of 1 lemon
- Juice of 1 lime
- 1 teaspoon extra-virgin olive oil
- 1 teaspoon ground cumin

1. In a blender or food processor, combine all the ingredients until smooth, adding chickpea liquid or water if necessary to blend, and create a creamy texture. Refrigerate until ready to serve. Serve with crunchy vegetables, crackers, or pita bread.

Per Serving:calorie: 56 / fat: 1g / protein: 3g / carbs: 9g / sugars: 2g / fiber: 2g / sodium: 76mg

Creamy Cheese Dip

Prep time: 5 minutes / Cook time: 5 minutes / Serves 40

- 1 cup plain fat-free yogurt, strained overnight in cheesecloth over a bowl set in the refrigerator
- 1 cup fat-free ricotta cheese
- 1 cup low-fat cottage cheese

1. Combine all the ingredients in a food processor; process until smooth. Place in a covered container, and refrigerate until ready to use (this cream cheese can be refrigerated for up to 1 week).

Per Serving:calorie: 21 / fat: 1g / protein: 2g / carbs: 1g / sugars: 1g / fiber: 0g / sodium: 81mg

Chilled Shrimp

Prep time: 5 minutes / Cook time: 5 minutes / Serves 20

- 5 pounds jumbo shrimp, unshelled
- ¼ cup plus 2 tablespoons extra-virgin olive oil, divided
- 4 medium lemons, thinly sliced
- 3 tablespoons minced garlic
- 3 medium red onions, thinly sliced
- ½ cup minced parsley
- Parsley sprigs (for garnish)

1. Preheat the oven to 400 degrees. Peel, and devein shrimp, leaving the tails intact.
2. Arrange the shrimp on a baking sheet and brush with 2 tablespoons of the olive oil. Bake the shrimp for 3 minutes or until they turn bright pink.
3. Place the lemon slices in a large bowl. Add the remaining ¼ cup of olive oil, garlic, onions, and minced parsley. Add the shrimp and toss vigorously to coat. Cover, and let marinate, refrigerated, for 6–8 hours.
4. Just before serving, arrange the shrimp on a serving platter. Garnish with parsley sprigs and some of the red onions and lemons from the bowl.

Per Serving:calorie: 127 / fat: 3g / protein: 23g / carbs: 2g / sugars: 0g / fiber: 0g / sodium: 136mg

Veggies with Cottage Cheese Ranch Dip

Prep time: 10 minutes / Cook time: 0 minutes / Serves 4

- 1 cup cottage cheese
- 2 tablespoons mayonnaise
- Juice of ½ lemon
- 2 tablespoons chopped fresh chives
- 2 tablespoons chopped fresh dill
- 2 scallions, white and green parts, finely chopped
- 1 garlic clove, minced
- ½ teaspoon sea salt
- 2 zucchinis, cut into sticks
- 8 cherry tomatoes

1. In a small bowl, mix the cottage cheese, mayonnaise, lemon juice, chives, dill, scallions, garlic, and salt.
2. Serve with the zucchini sticks and cherry tomatoes for dipping.

Per Serving:calorie: 88 / fat: 3g / protein: 6g / carbs: 10g / sugars: 4g / fiber: 2g / sodium: 495mg

Guacamole

Prep time: 5 minutes / Cook time: 5 minutes / Serves 8

- 2 large (8½ ounces) ripe avocados, peeled, pits removed, and mashed
- ½ cup chopped onion
- 2 medium jalapeño peppers, seeded and chopped
- 2 tablespoons minced fresh parsley
- 2 tablespoons fresh lime juice
- ⅛ teaspoon freshly ground black pepper
- 2 medium tomatoes, fincly chopped
- 1 medium garlic clove, minced
- 1 tablespoon extra-virgin olive oil
- ½ teaspoon salt

1. In a large mixing bowl, combine all ingredients, blending well.

Per Serving:calorie: 107 / fat: 9g / protein: 1g / carbs: 7g / sugars: 2g / fiber: 4g / sodium: 152mg

Lemon Cream Fruit Dip

Prep time: 5 minutes / Cook time: 0 minutes / Serves 4

- 1 cup (200 g) plain nonfat Greek yogurt
- ¼ cup (28 g) coconut flour 1 tablespoon (15 ml) pure maple syrup
- ½ teaspoon pure vanilla extract
- ½ teaspoon pure almond extract
- Zest of 1 medium lemon
- Juice of ½ medium lemon

1. In a medium bowl, whisk together the yogurt, coconut flour, maple syrup, vanilla, almond extract, lemon zest, and lemon juice. Serve the dip with fruit or crackers.

Per Serving:calorie: 80 / fat: 1g / protein: 7g / carbs: 10g / sugars: 6g / fiber: 3g / sodium: 37mg

Gruyere Apple Spread

Prep time: 5 minutes / Cook time: 5 minutes / Serves 20

- 4 ounces fat-free cream cheese, softened
- ½ cup low-fat cottage cheese
- 4 ounces Gruyere cheese
- ¼ teaspoon dry mustard
- ⅛ teaspoon freshly ground black pepper
- ½ cup shredded apple (unpeeled)
- 2 tablespoons finely chopped pecans
- 2 teaspoons minced fresh chives

1. Place the cheeses in a food processor, and blend until smooth. Add the mustard and pepper, and blend for 30 seconds.
2. Transfer the mixture to a serving bowl, and fold in the apple and pecans. Sprinkle the dip with chives.
3. Cover, and refrigerate the mixture for 1–2 hours. Serve chilled with crackers, or stuff into celery stalks.

Per Serving:calorie: 46 / fat: 3g / protein: 4g / carbs: 1g / sugars: 1g / fiber: 0g / sodium: 107mg

Monterey Jack Cheese Quiche Squares

Prep time: 10 minutes / Cook time: 15 minutes / Serves 12

- 4 egg whites
- 1 cup plus 2 tablespoons low-fat cottage cheese
- ¼ cup plus 2 tablespoons flour
- ¾ teaspoon baking powder
- 1 cup shredded reduced-fat Monterey Jack cheese
- ½ cup diced green chilies
- 1 red bell pepper, diced
- 1 cup lentils, cooked
- 1 tablespoon extra-virgin olive oil
- Parsley sprigs

1. Preheat the oven to 350 degrees.
2. In a medium bowl, beat the egg whites and cottage cheese for 2 minutes, until smooth.
3. Add the flour and baking powder, and beat until smooth. Stir in the cheese, green chilies, red pepper, and lentils.
4. Coat a 9-inch-square pan with the olive oil, and pour in the egg mixture. Bake for 30–35 minutes, until firm.
5. Remove the quiche from the oven, and allow to cool for 10 minutes (it will be easier to cut). Cut into 12 squares and transfer to a platter, garnish with parsley sprigs, and serve.

Per Serving:calorie: 104 / fat: 6g / protein: 8g / carbs: 4g / sugars: 0g / fiber: 0g / sodium: 215mg

Lemony White Bean Puree

Prep time: 10 minutes / Cook time: 0 minutes / Makes 4 cups

- 1 (15-ounce) can white beans, drained and rinsed
- 1 small onion, coarsely chopped
- 1 garlic clove, minced
- Zest and juice of 1 lemon
- ½ teaspoon herbs de Provence
- 3 tablespoons extra-virgin olive oil, divided
- 1 tablespoon chopped fresh parsley

1. Place the beans, onion, garlic, lemon zest and juice, and herbs in a food processor and pulse until smooth. While the machine is running, slowly stream in 2 tablespoons of extra-virgin olive oil. If the mixture is too thick, add water very slowly until you've reached the desired consistency.
2. Transfer the puree to a medium serving bowl. Top with the remaining 1 tablespoon of extra-virgin olive oil and the parsley.
3. Serve with your favorite vegetable or flatbread of choice. Store any leftovers in an airtight container in the refrigerator for up to 4 days.

Per Serving:calorie: 121 / fat: 5g / protein: 5g / carbs: 15g / sugars: 1g / fiber: 3g / sodium: 4mg

Hummus with Chickpeas and Tahini Sauce

Prep time: 10 minutes / Cook time: 55 minutes / Makes 4 cups

- 4 cups water
- 1 cup dried chickpeas
- 2½ teaspoons fine sea salt
- ½ cup tahini
- 3 tablespoons fresh lemon juice
- 1 garlic clove
- ¼ teaspoon ground cumin

1. Combine the water, chickpeas, and 1 teaspoon of the salt in the Instant Pot and stir to dissolve the salt.
2. Secure the lid and set the Pressure Release to Sealing. Select the Bean/Chili, Pressure Cook, or

Manual setting and set the cooking time for 40 minutes at high pressure. (The pot will take about 15 minutes to come up to pressure before the cooking program begins.)

3. When the cooking program ends, let the pressure release naturally for 15 minutes, then move the Pressure Release to Venting to release any remaining steam.

4. Place a colander over a bowl. Open the pot and, wearing heat-resistant mitts, lift out the inner pot and drain the beans in the colander. Return the chickpeas to the inner pot and place it back in the Instant Pot housing on the Keep Warm setting. Reserve the cooking liquid.

5. In a blender or food processor, combine 1 cup of the cooking liquid, the tahini, lemon juice, garlic, cumin, and 1 teaspoon salt. Blend or process on high speed, stopping to scrape down the sides of the container as needed, for about 30 seconds, until smooth and a little fluffy. Scoop out and set aside ½ cup of this sauce for the topping.

6. Set aside ½ cup of the chickpeas for the topping. Add the remaining chickpeas to the tahini sauce in the blender or food processor along with ½ cup of the cooking liquid and the remaining ½ teaspoon salt. Blend or process on high speed, stopping to scrape down the sides of the container as needed, for about 1 minute, until very smooth.

7. Transfer the hummus to a shallow serving bowl. Spoon the reserved tahini mixture over the top, then sprinkle on the reserved chickpeas. The hummus will keep in an airtight container in the refrigerator for up to 3 days. Serve at room temperature or chilled.

Per Serving:calories: 107 / fat: 5g / protein: 4g / carbs: 10g / sugars: 3g / fiber: 4g / sodium: 753mg

Baked Scallops

Prep time: 5 minutes / Cook time: 10 minutes / Serves 4

- 12 ounces fresh bay or dry sea scallops
- 1½ teaspoons salt-free pickling spices
- ½ cup cider vinegar
- ¼ cup water
- 1 tablespoon finely chopped onion
- 1 red bell pepper, cut into thin strips
- 1 head butter lettuce, rinsed and dried
- ⅓ cup sesame seeds, toasted

1. Preheat the oven to 350 degrees. Wash the scallops in cool water, and cut any scallops that are too big in half.

2. Spread the scallops out in a large baking dish (be careful not to overlap them). In a small bowl, combine the spices, cider vinegar, water, onion, and pepper; pour the mixture over the scallops.

Season with salt, if desired.

3. Cover the baking dish and bake for 7 minutes. Remove from the oven, and allow the scallops to chill in the refrigerator (leave them in the cooking liquid/vegetable mixture).

4. Just before serving, place the lettuce leaves on individual plates or a platter, and place the scallops and vegetables over the top. Sprinkle with sesame seeds before serving.

Per Serving:calorie: 159 / fat: 8g / protein: 14g / carbs: 7g / sugars: 2g / fiber: 3g / sodium: 344mg

Zucchini Hummus Dip with Red Bell Peppers

Prep time: 10 minutes / Cook time: 0 minutes / Serves 4

- 2 zucchini, chopped
- 3 garlic cloves
- 2 tablespoons extra-virgin olive oil
- 2 tablespoons tahini
- Juice of 1 lemon
- ½ teaspoon sea salt
- 1 red bell pepper, seeded and cut into sticks

1. In a blender or food processor, combine the zucchini, garlic, olive oil, tahini, lemon juice, and salt. Blend until smooth.

2. Serve with the red bell pepper for dipping.

Per Serving:calorie: 136 / fat: 11g / protein: 3g / carbs: 8g / sugars: 4g / fiber: 2g / sodium: 309mg

Roasted Carrot and Herb Spread

Prep time: 20 minutes / Cook time: 1 hour / Serves 16

- 1 pound ready-to-eat baby-cut carrots
- 1 dark orange sweet potato, peeled, cut into 1-inch pieces (2½ cups)
- 1 small onion, cut into 8 wedges, separated
- 2 tablespoons olive oil
- 1 clove garlic, finely chopped
- 1 tablespoon chopped fresh or 1 teaspoon dried thyme leaves
- ¼ teaspoon salt
- ⅛ teaspoon freshly ground pepper
- Assorted whole-grain crackers or vegetable chips

1. Heat oven to 350°F. Spray 15x10x1-inch pan with cooking spray. Place carrots, sweet potato and onion in pan; drizzle with oil. Sprinkle with garlic, thyme, salt and pepper; stir to coat.

2. Bake uncovered about 1 hour, stirring occasionally, until vegetables are tender.

3. In food processor, place vegetable mixture. Cover; process until blended. Spoon into serving bowl. Serve warm, or cover and refrigerate until serving. Serve with crackers.

Per Serving:calories: 90 / fat: 4g / protein: 1g / carbs: 12g / sugars: 3g / fiber: 2g / sodium: 125mg

Chapter 7 Vegetables and Sides

Ribboned Squash with Bacon

Prep time: 15 minutes / Cook time: 10 minutes / Serves 4

- ¼ cup dried currants or golden raisins
- ¼ cup red wine vinegar
- 1 pound butternut squash, seeded and skin removed
- 4 bacon slices
- 2 tablespoons extra-virgin olive oil (optional)
- ½ cup chopped, toasted walnuts
- 4 cups arugula
- Freshly ground black pepper
- ½ cup chopped fresh parsley

1. In a small bowl, combine the currants and vinegar and allow to soak until tender, about 10 minutes.
2. Using a vegetable peeler, peel the squash into long ribbons into a large bowl. Set aside.
3. Place the bacon slices in a medium skillet over medium heat, cover, and fry for 8 to 10 minutes until cooked through and crispy. Remove the bacon from the heat and drain it on a paper towel. Chop the bacon into bite-size pieces when it's cool enough to handle.
4. Return the pan to medium heat with the bacon fat (or wipe it out and then add the extra-virgin olive oil). Add the walnuts. Heat the walnuts for 2 minutes, then transfer the mixture from the skillet to the squash noodles and toss well. Add the currants with their soaking liquid, along with the arugula and reserved bacon.
5. Season with pepper and serve topped with parsley.
6. Store any leftovers in an airtight container in the refrigerator for up to 4 days.

Per Serving:calories: 294 / fat: 24g / protein: 7g / carbs: 16g / sugars: 3g / fiber: 4g / sodium: 138mg

Vegetable Curry

Prep time: 25 minutes / Cook time: 3 minutes / Serves 10

- 16-ounce package baby carrots
- 3 medium potatoes, unpeeled, cubed
- 1 pound fresh or frozen green beans, cut in 2-inch pieces
- 1 medium green pepper, chopped
- 1 medium onion, chopped
- 1–2 cloves garlic, minced
- 15-ounce can garbanzo beans, drained
- 28-ounce can crushed tomatoes
- 3 teaspoons curry powder
- 1½ teaspoons chicken bouillon granules
- 1¾ cups boiling water
- 3 tablespoons minute tapioca

1. Combine carrots, potatoes, green beans, pepper, onion, garlic, garbanzo beans, crushed tomatoes, and curry powder in the Instant Pot.
2. Dissolve bouillon in boiling water, then stir in tapicoa. Pour over the contents of the Instant Pot and stir.
3. Secure the lid and make sure vent is set to sealing. Press Manual and set for 3 minutes.
4. When cook time is up, manually release the pressure.

Per Serving:calories: 166 / fat: 1g / protein: 6g / carbs: 35g / sugars: 10g / fiber: 8g / sodium: 436mg

Green Beans with Garlic and Onion

Prep time: 5 minutes / Cook time: 12 minutes / Serves 8

- 1 pound fresh green beans, trimmed and cut into 2-inch pieces
- 1 tablespoon extra-virgin olive oil
- 1 small onion, chopped
- 1 large garlic clove, minced
- 1 tablespoon white vinegar
- ¼ cup Parmigiano-Reggiano cheese
- ⅛ teaspoon freshly ground black pepper

1. Steam the beans for 7 minutes or until just tender. Set aside.
2. In a skillet, heat the oil over low heat. Add the onion and garlic, and sauté for 4–5 minutes or until the onion is translucent.
3. Transfer the beans to a serving bowl, and add the onion mixture and vinegar, tossing well. Sprinkle with cheese and pepper, and serve.

Per Serving:calories: 43 / fat: 3g / protein: 1g / carbs: 4g / sugars: 1g / fiber: 1g / sodium: 30mg

Italian Wild Mushrooms

Prep time: 30 minutes / Cook time: 3 minutes / Serves 10

- 2 tablespoons canola oil
- 2 large onions, chopped
- 4 garlic cloves, minced
- 3 large red bell peppers, chopped
- 3 large green bell peppers, chopped
- 12 ounces package oyster mushrooms, cleaned and chopped
- 3 fresh bay leaves
- 10 fresh basil leaves, chopped
- 1 teaspoon salt
- 1½ teaspoons pepper
- 28 ounces can Italian plum tomatoes, crushed or chopped

1. Press Sauté on the Instant Pot and add in the oil. Once the oil is heated, add the onions, garlic, peppers, and mushroom to the oil. Sauté just until mushrooms begin to turn brown.

2. Add remaining ingredients. Stir well.
3. Secure the lid and make sure vent is set to sealing. Press Manual and set time for 3 minutes.
4. When cook time is up, release the pressure manually. Discard bay leaves.

Per Serving:calories: 82 / fat: 3g / protein: 3g / carbs: 13g / sugars: 8g / fiber: 4g / sodium: 356mg

Teriyaki Chickpeas

Prep time: 5 minutes / Cook time: 20 to 25 minutes / Serves 7

• 2 cans (15 ounces each) chickpeas, rinsed and drained
• 1½ tablespoons tamari
• 1 tablespoon pure maple syrup
• 1 tablespoon lemon juice
• ½ to ¾ teaspoon garlic powder
• ½ teaspoon ground ginger
• ½ teaspoon blackstrap molasses

1. Preheat the oven to 450°F. Line a baking sheet with parchment paper.
2. In a large mixing bowl, combine the chickpeas, tamari, syrup, lemon juice, garlic powder, ginger, and molasses. Toss to combine. Spread evenly on the prepared baking sheet and bake for 20 to 25 minutes, or until the marinade is absorbed. Serve warm, or refrigerate to enjoy later.

Per Serving:calorie: 120 / fat: 2 / protein: 6g / carbs: 20g / sugars: 5g / fiber: 5g / sodium: 382mg

Pico de Gallo Navy Beans

Prep time: 20 minutes / Cook time: 0 minutes / Serves 4

• 2½ cups cooked navy beans   • 1 tomato, diced
• ½ red bell pepper, seeded and chopped
• ¼ jalapeño pepper, chopped
• 1 scallion, white and green parts, chopped
• 1 teaspoon minced garlic
• 1 teaspoon ground cumin
• ½ teaspoon ground coriander
• ½ cup low-sodium feta cheese

1. Put the beans, tomato, bell pepper, jalapeño, scallion, garlic, cumin, and coriander in a medium bowl and stir until well mixed.
2. Top with the feta cheese and serve.

Per Serving:calories: 218 / fat: 4g / protein: 14g / carbs: 33g / sugars: 2g / fiber: 13g / sodium: 6mg

Avocado Slaw

Prep time: 15 minutes / Cook time: 0 minutes / Serves 4 to 6

• 1 avocado   • ⅓ cup water
• 3 tablespoons apple cider vinegar
• 1 tablespoon Dijon mustard
• 4 cups packed shredded cabbage (red, green, or mixed)
• 2 cups shredded carrot

• Kosher salt
• Freshly ground black pepper

1. Place the avocado, water, vinegar, and mustard in a blender and puree until smooth. Add water if needed until you've reached a thin consistency, making the dressing easy to toss with the shredded vegetables.
2. In a large bowl, toss the cabbage and carrot with the dressing. Season to taste with salt and pepper and serve.
3. Store any leftovers in an airtight container in the refrigerator for up to 3 days.

Per Serving:calories: 137 / fat: 8g / protein: 2g / carbs: 17g / sugars: 6g / fiber: 7g / sodium: 400mg

Sautéed Spinach and Tomatoes

Prep time: 5 minutes / Cook time: 10 minutes / Serves 4

• 1 tablespoon extra-virgin olive oil
• 1 cup cherry tomatoes, halved
• 3 spinach bunches, trimmed
• 2 garlic cloves, minced   • ¼ teaspoon salt

1. In a large skillet, heat the oil over medium heat.
2. Add the tomatoes, and cook until the skins begin to blister and split, about 2 minutes.
3. Add the spinach in batches, waiting for each batch to wilt slightly before adding the next batch. Stir continuously for 3 to 4 minutes until the spinach is tender.
4. Add the garlic to the skillet, and toss until fragrant, about 30 seconds.
5. Drain the excess liquid from the pan. Add the salt. Stir well and serve.

Per Serving:calories: 52 / fat: 4g / protein: 2g / carbs: 4g / sugars: 1g / fiber: 2g / sodium: 183mg

Garlicky Cabbage and Collard Greens

Prep time: 10 minutes / Cook time: 10 minutes / Serves 8

• 2 tablespoons extra-virgin olive oil
• 1 collard greens bunch, stemmed and thinly sliced
• ½ small green cabbage, thinly sliced
• 6 garlic cloves, minced
• 1 tablespoon low-sodium gluten-free soy sauce or tamari

1. In a large skillet, heat the oil over medium-high heat.
2. Add the collards to the pan, stirring to coat with oil. Sauté for 1 to 2 minutes until the greens begin to wilt.
3. Add the cabbage and stir to coat. Cover and reduce the heat to medium low. Continue to cook for 5 to 7 minutes, stirring once or twice, until the greens are tender.
4. Add the garlic and soy sauce and stir to incorporate. Cook until just fragrant, about 30 seconds longer.

Serve warm and enjoy!

Per Serving:calories: 72/ fat: 4g / protein: 3g / carbs: 6g / sugars: 0g / fiber: 3g / sodium: 129mg

Lemon-Garlic Mushrooms

Prep time: 10 minutes / Cook time: 10 to 15 minutes / Serves 6

- 12 ounces (340 g) sliced mushrooms
- 1 tablespoon avocado oil
- Sea salt and freshly ground black pepper, to taste
- 3 tablespoons unsalted butter
- 1 teaspoon minced garlic
- 1 teaspoon freshly squeezed lemon juice
- ½ teaspoon red pepper flakes
- 2 tablespoons chopped fresh parsley

1. Place the mushrooms in a medium bowl and toss with the oil. Season to taste with salt and pepper.
2. Place the mushrooms in a single layer in the air fryer basket. Set your air fryer to 375°F (191ºC) and roast for 10 to 15 minutes, until the mushrooms are tender.
3. While the mushrooms cook, melt the butter in a small pot or skillet over medium-low heat. Stir in the garlic and cook for 30 seconds. Remove the pot from the heat and stir in the lemon juice and red pepper flakes.
4. Toss the mushrooms with the lemon-garlic butter and garnish with the parsley before serving.

Per Serving:calorie: 90 / fat: 7g / protein: 2g / carbs: 6g / sugars: 2g / fiber: 2g / sodium: 70mg

Brussels Sprouts with Pecans and Gorgonzola

Prep time: 10 minutes / Cook time: 25 minutes / Serves 4

- ½ cup pecans
- 1½ pounds (680 g) fresh Brussels sprouts, trimmed and quartered
- 2 tablespoons olive oil
- Salt and freshly ground black pepper, to taste
- ¼ cup crumbled Gorgonzola cheese

1. Spread the pecans in a single layer of the air fryer and set the heat to 350ºF (177ºC). Air fry for 3 to 5 minutes until the pecans are lightly browned and fragrant. Transfer the pecans to a plate and continue preheating the air fryer, increasing the heat to 400ºF (204ºC).
2. In a large bowl, toss the Brussels sprouts with the olive oil and season with salt and black pepper to taste.
3. Working in batches if necessary, arrange the Brussels sprouts in a single layer in the air fryer basket. Pausing halfway through the baking time to shake the basket, air fry for 20 to 25 minutes until the sprouts are tender and starting to brown on the edges.
4. Transfer the sprouts to a serving bowl and top with

the toasted pecans and Gorgonzola. Serve warm or at room temperature.

Per Serving:calorie: 280 / fat: 22g / protein: 8g / carbs: 17g / sugars: 5g / fiber: 7g / sodium: 310mg

Asparagus with Cashews

Prep time: 10 minutes / Cook time: 20 minutes / Serves 4

- 1 tablespoon extra-virgin olive oil
- Sea salt   • Freshly ground black pepper
- ½ cup chopped cashews
- Zest and juice of 1 lime

1. Preheat the oven to 400°F and line a baking sheet with aluminum foil.
2. In a large bowl, toss the asparagus with the oil and lightly season with salt and pepper.
3. Transfer the asparagus to the baking sheet and bake until tender and lightly browned, 15 to 20 minutes.
4. Transfer the asparagus to a serving bowl and toss them with the chopped cashews, lime zest, and lime juice.

Per Serving:calories: 123 / fat: 11g / protein: 3g / carbs: 6g / sugars: 1g / fiber: 1g / sodium: 148mg

Spicy Roasted Cauliflower with Lime

Prep time: 5 minutes / Cook time: 10 minutes / Serves 4

- 1 cauliflower head, broken into small florets
- 2 tablespoons extra-virgin olive oil
- ½ teaspoon ground chipotle chili powder
- ½ teaspoon salt   • Juice of 1 lime

1. Preheat the oven to 450°F. Line a rimmed baking sheet with parchment paper.
2. In a large mixing bowl, toss the cauliflower with the olive oil, chipotle chili powder, and salt. Arrange in a single layer on the prepared baking sheet.
3. Roast for 15 minutes, flip, and continue to roast for 15 more minutes until well-browned and tender.
4. Sprinkle with the lime juice, adjust the salt as needed, and serve.

Per Serving:calories: 99 / fat: 7 / protein: 3g / carbs: 8g / sugars: 3g / fiber: 3g / sodium: 284mg

Fried Zucchini Salad

Prep time: 10 minutes / Cook time: 5 to 7 minutes / Serves 4

- 2 medium zucchini, thinly sliced
- 5 tablespoons olive oil, divided
- ¼ cup chopped fresh parsley
- 2 tablespoons chopped fresh mint
- Zest and juice of ½ lemon
- 1 clove garlic, minced
- ¼ cup crumbled feta cheese
- Freshly ground black pepper, to taste

1. Preheat the air fryer to 400°F (204°C).
2. In a large bowl, toss the zucchini slices with 1 tablespoon of the olive oil.
3. Working in batches if necessary, arrange the zucchini slices in an even layer in the air fryer basket. Pausing halfway through the cooking time to shake the basket, air fry for 5 to 7 minutes until soft and lightly browned on each side.
4. Meanwhile, in a small bowl, combine the remaining 4 tablespoons olive oil, parsley, mint, lemon zest, lemon juice, and garlic.
5. Arrange the zucchini on a plate and drizzle with the dressing. Sprinkle the feta and black pepper on top. Serve warm or at room temperature.

Per Serving:calories: 190 / fat: 19g / protein: 3g / carbs: 4g / sugars: 2g / fiber: 1g / sodium: 131mg

Snow Peas with Sesame Seeds

Prep time: 5 minutes / Cook time: 5 minutes / Serves 6

• 2 cups water
• 1 pound trimmed fresh snow peas
• 3 tablespoons sesame seeds
• 1 tablespoon chopped shallots
• ¼ teaspoon salt
• ⅛ teaspoon freshly ground black pepper
• 1 teaspoon ground ginger

1. In a saucepan over high heat, boil the water. Add the snow peas, and then turn off the heat. After 1 minute, rinse the snow peas under cold running water to stop the cooking process; drain. (This method of blanching helps the snow peas to retain their bright green color and crispness.)
2. In a skillet, toast the sesame seeds for 1 minute over medium heat. Add the snow peas, shallots, salt, pepper, and ginger. Continue sautéing for 1–2 minutes until the snow peas are coated with sesame seeds. Serve.

Per Serving:calories: 59 / fat: 3g / protein: 3g / carbs: 7g / sugars: 3g / fiber: 3g / sodium: 104mg

Spaghetti Squash

Prep time: 5 minutes / Cook time: 7 minutes / Serves 4

• 1 spaghetti squash (about 2 pounds)

1. Cut the spaghetti squash in half crosswise and use a large spoon to remove the seeds.
2. Pour 1 cup of water into the electric pressure cooker and insert a wire rack or trivet.
3. Place the squash halves on the rack, cut-side up.
4. Close and lock the lid of the pressure cooker. Set the valve to sealing.
5. Cook on high pressure for 7 minutes.
6. When the cooking is complete, hit Cancel and

quick release the pressure.
7. Once the pin drops, unlock and remove the lid.
8. With tongs, remove the squash from the pot and transfer it to a plate. When it is cool enough to handle, scrape the squash with the tines of a fork to remove the strands. Discard the skin.

Per Serving:calories: 121 / fat: 2g / protein: 2g / carbs: 28g / sugars: 11g / fiber: 6g / sodium: 68mg

Dandelion Greens with Sweet Onion

Prep time: 15 minutes / Cook time: 15 minutes / Serves 4

• 1 tablespoon extra-virgin olive oil
• 1 Vidalia onion, thinly sliced
• 2 garlic cloves, minced
• ½ cup store-bought low-sodium vegetable broth
• 2 bunches dandelion greens, roughly chopped
• Freshly ground black pepper

1. In a large skillet, heat the olive oil over low heat.
2. Add the onion and garlic and cook, stirring to prevent the garlic from scorching, for 2 to 3 minutes, or until the onion is translucent.
3. Add the broth and greens and cook, stirring often, for 5 to 7 minutes, or until the greens are wilted.
4. Season with pepper, and serve warm.

Per Serving:calories: 53 / fat: 4g / protein: 1g / carbs: 5g / sugars: 1g / fiber: 1g / sodium: 39mg

Sautéed Mixed Vegetables

Prep time: 20 minutes / Cook time: 8 minutes / Serves 4

• 2 teaspoons extra-virgin olive oil
• 2 carrots, peeled and sliced
• 4 cups broccoli florets • 4 cups cauliflower florets
• 1 red bell pepper, seeded and cut into long strips
• 1 cup green beans, trimmed   • Sea salt
• Freshly ground black pepper

1. Place a large skillet over medium heat and add the olive oil.
2. Sauté the carrots, broccoli, and cauliflower until tender-crisp, about 6 minutes.
3. Add the bell pepper and green beans, and sauté 2 minutes more.
4. Season with salt and pepper, and serve.

Per Serving:calories: 97 / fat: 3g / protein: 5g / carbs: 15g / sugars: 5g / fiber: 6g / sodium: 211mg

Sweet Potato Crisps

Prep time: 10 minutes / Cook time: 30 minutes / Serves 3

• 1 pound sweet potatoes
• ½ tablespoon balsamic vinegar
• ½ tablespoon pure maple syrup
• Rounded ¼ teaspoon sea salt

1. Preheat the oven to 400°F. Line a large baking

sheet with parchment paper.

2. Peel the sweet potatoes, then use the peeler to continue to make sweet potato peelings. (Alternatively, you can push peeled sweet potatoes through a food processor slicing blade.) Transfer the peelings to a large mixing bowl and use your hands to toss with the vinegar and syrup, coating them as evenly as possible. Spread the peelings on the prepared baking sheet, spacing well. Sprinkle with the salt. Bake for 30 minutes, tossing once or twice. The pieces around the edges of the pan can get brown quickly, so move the chips around during baking. Turn off the oven and let the chips sit in the residual heat for 20 minutes, stir again, and let sit for another 15 to 20 minutes, until they crisp up. Remove, and snack!

Per Serving:calorie: 94 / fat: 0g / protein: 2g / carbs: 22g / sugars: 8g / fiber: 3g / sodium: 326mg

Summer Squash Casserole

Prep time: 15 minutes / Cook time: 30 minutes / Serves 8

- 1 tablespoon extra-virgin olive oil
- 6 yellow summer squash, thinly sliced
- 1 large portobello mushroom, thinly sliced
- 1 Vidalia onion, thinly sliced
- 1 cup shredded Parmesan cheese, divided
- 1 cup shredded reduced-fat extra-sharp Cheddar cheese
- ½ cup whole-wheat bread crumbs
- ½ cup tri-color quinoa
- 1 tablespoon Creole seasoning

1. Preheat the oven to 350°F.
2. In a large cast iron pan, heat the oil over medium heat.
3. Add the squash, mushroom, and onion, and sauté for 7 to 10 minutes, or until softened.
4. Remove from the heat. Add ½ cup of Parmesan cheese and the Cheddar cheese and mix well.
5. In a small bowl, whisk the bread crumbs, quinoa, the remaining ½ cup of Parmesan, and the Creole seasoning together. Evenly distribute over the casserole.
6. Transfer the pan to the oven, and bake for 20 minutes, or until browned. Serve warm and enjoy.

Per Serving:calories: 163 / fat: 7g / protein: 10g / carbs: 14g / sugars: 1g / fiber: 2g / sodium: 484mg

Wild Rice Salad with Cranberries and Almonds

Prep time: 10 minutes / Cook time: 25 minutes / Serves 18

- For the rice
- 2 cups wild rice blend, rinsed
- 1 teaspoon kosher salt
- 2½ cups Vegetable Broth or Chicken Bone Broth
- For the dressing

- ¼ cup extra-virgin olive oil
- ¼ cup white wine vinegar
- 1½ teaspoons grated orange zest
- Juice of 1 medium orange (about ¼ cup)
- 1 teaspoon honey or pure maple syrup
- For the salad
- ¾ cup unsweetened dried cranberries
- ½ cup sliced almonds, toasted
- Freshly ground black pepper

Make the Rice 1. In the electric pressure cooker, combine the rice, salt, and broth.

2. Close and lock the lid. Set the valve to sealing.
3. Cook on high pressure for 25 minutes.
4. When the cooking is complete, hit Cancel and allow the pressure to release naturally for 15 minutes, then quick release any remaining pressure.
5. Once the pin drops, unlock and remove the lid.
6. Let the rice cool briefly, then fluff it with a fork. Make the Dressing 7. While the rice cooks, make the dressing: In a small jar with a screw-top lid, combine the olive oil, vinegar, zest, juice, and honey. (If you don't have a jar, whisk the ingredients together in a small bowl.) Shake to combine. Make the Salad 8. In a large bowl, combine the rice, cranberries, and almonds.
9. Add the dressing and season with pepper.
10. Serve warm or refrigerate.

Per Serving:calories: 129 / fat: 4g / protein: 3g / carbs: 20g / sugars: 5g / fiber: 2g / sodium: 200mg

Roasted Beets, Carrots, and Parsnips

Prep time: 10 minutes / Cook time: 30 minutes / Serves 4

- 1 pound beets, peeled and quartered
- ½ pound carrots, peeled and cut into chunks
- ½ pound parsnips, peeled and cut into chunks
- 1 tablespoon extra-virgin olive oil
- 1 teaspoon apple cider vinegar
- Sea salt
- Freshly ground black pepper

1. Preheat the oven to 375°F. Line a baking tray with aluminum foil.
2. In a large bowl, toss the beets, carrots, and parsnips with the oil and vinegar until everything is well coated. Spread them out on the baking sheet.
3. Roast until the vegetables are tender and lightly caramelized, about 30 minutes.
4. Transfer the vegetables to a serving bowl, season with salt and pepper, and serve warm.

Per Serving:calories: 122 / fat: 4g / protein: 4g / carbs: 21g / sugars: 6g / fiber: 9g / sodium: 592mg

Asparagus with Vinaigrette

Prep time: 5 minutes / Cook time: 10 minutes / Serves 6

- 1½ pounds fresh or frozen asparagus (thin pieces)
- ½ cup red wine vinegar
- ½ teaspoon dried or 1 teaspoon fresh tarragon
- 2 tablespoons finely chopped fresh chives
- 3 tablespoons finely chopped fresh parsley
- ½ cup water
- 1 tablespoon extra-virgin olive oil
- 1⅓ tablespoons Dijon mustard
- 1 pound fresh spinach leaves, trimmed of stems, washed, and dried
- 2 large tomatoes, cut into wedges

1. Place 1 inch of water in a pot, and place a steamer inside. Arrange the asparagus on top of the steamer. Steam fresh asparagus for 4 minutes or frozen asparagus for 6–8 minutes. Immediately rinse the asparagus under cold water to stop the cooking. (This helps keep asparagus bright green and crunchy.) Set aside.
2. In a small bowl or salad cruet, combine the remaining ingredients except the spinach and tomatoes. Mix, or shake well.
3. To serve, line plates with the spinach leaves, and place the asparagus on top of the spinach. Garnish with the tomato wedges, and spoon any remaining dressing on top.

Per Serving:calories: 72 / fat: 2g / protein: 7g / carbs: 10g / sugars: 2g / fiber: 5g / sodium: 133mg

Simple Bibimbap

Prep time: 15 minutes / Cook time: 15 minutes / Serves 2

- 4 teaspoons canola oil, divided
- 2½ cups cauliflower rice• 2 cups fresh baby spinach
- 3 teaspoons low-sodium soy sauce or tamari, divided
- 8 ounces mushrooms, thinly sliced
- 2 large eggs   • 1 cup bean sprouts, rinsed
- 1 cup kimchi   • ½ cup shredded carrots

1. Heat 1 teaspoon of canola oil in a medium skillet and sauté the cauliflower rice, spinach, and 2 teaspoons of soy sauce until the greens are wilted, about 5 minutes. Put the vegetables in a small bowl and set aside.
2. Return the skillet to medium heat, add 2 teaspoons of vegetable oil and, when it's hot, add the mushrooms in a single layer and cook for 3 to 5 minutes, then stir and cook another 3 minutes or until mostly golden-brown in color. Put the mushrooms in a small bowl and toss them with the remaining 1 teaspoon of soy sauce.
3. Wipe out the skillet and heat the remaining 1 teaspoon of vegetable oil over low heat. Crack in the eggs and cook until the whites are set and the yolks begin to thicken but not harden, 4 to 5 minutes.
4. Assemble two bowls with cauliflower rice and spinach at the bottom. Then arrange each

ingredient separately around the rim of the bowl: bean sprouts, mushrooms, kimchi, and shredded carrots, with the egg placed in the center, and serve.

Per Serving:calories: 275 / fat: 16g / protein: 20g / carbs: 20g / sugars: 8g / fiber: 8g / sodium: 518mg

Green Bean and Radish Potato Salad

Prep time: 10 minutes / Cook time: 20 minutes / Serves 6

- Kosher salt
- 6 ounces fresh green beans, trimmed and cut into 1-inch pieces
- 1½ pounds fingerling potatoes
- ⅓ cup extra-virgin olive oil
- 2 tablespoons freshly squeezed lemon juice
- 1 tablespoon Dijon or whole-grain mustard
- 1 shallot, minced   • 8 radishes, thinly sliced
- ¼ cup fresh dill, chopped
- Freshly ground black pepper

1. Place a small saucepan filled three-quarters full of water and a pinch of salt over high heat and bring it to a boil. Add the green beans and boil for 2 minutes, then transfer them with a slotted spoon to a colander. Run the beans under cold running water until cool and transfer to a medium bowl.
2. Place the potatoes in the same pot of boiling water, reduce the heat to low, and simmer until tender, about 12 minutes.
3. Meanwhile, combine the extra-virgin olive oil, lemon juice, mustard, and shallot in a jar. Seal with the lid and shake vigorously. If you don't have a jar with a fitted lid, you can also whisk the ingredients in a bowl.
4. Transfer the cooked potatoes to a colander and cool them under cold running water. When they're cool enough to handle, slice the potatoes into thin rounds.
5. Add the potatoes and dressing to the bowl with the green beans, along with the radishes and dill, and toss to combine.
6. Season with salt and pepper and serve.
7. Store any leftovers in an airtight container in the refrigerator for 3 to 4 days.

Per Serving:calories: 206 / fat: 12g / protein: 3g / carbs: 23g / sugars: 1g / fiber: 3g / sodium: 202mg

Nutmeg Green Beans

Prep time: 15 minutes / Cook time: 5 minutes / Serves 12

- 1 tablespoon butter
- 1½ pounds green beans, trimmed
- 1 teaspoon ground nutmeg   • Sea salt

1. Place a large skillet over medium heat and melt the butter.
2. Add the green beans and sauté, stirring often, until the beans are tender-crisp, about 5 minutes.

3. Stir in the nutmeg and season with salt.
4. Serve immediately.

Per Serving:calories: 22 / fat: 1g / protein: 1g / carbs: 3g / sugars: 0g / fiber: 1g / sodium: 57mg

Spaghetti Squash with Sun-Dried Tomatoes

Prep time: 20 minutes / Cook time: 1hour / Serves 4

- 1 spaghetti squash, halved and seeded
- 3 teaspoons extra-virgin olive oil, divided
- ¼ sweet onion, chopped
- 1 teaspoon minced garlic
- 2 cups fresh spinach
- ¼ cup chopped sun-dried tomatoes
- ¼ cup roasted, shelled sunflower seeds
- Juice of ½ lemon   • Sea salt
- Freshly ground black pepper

1. Preheat the oven to 350°F. Line a baking sheet with parchment paper.
2. Place the squash on the baking sheet and brush the cut edges with 2 teaspoons of olive oil.
3. Bake the squash until it is tender and separates into strands with a fork, about 1 hour.
4. Let the squash cool for 5 minutes then use a fork to scrape out the strands from both halves of the squash. Cover the squash strands and set them aside.
5. Place a large skillet over medium-high heat and add the remaining 1 teaspoon of olive oil. Sauté the onion and garlic until softened and translucent, about 3 minutes.
6. Stir in the spinach and sun-dried tomatoes, and sauté until the spinach is wilted, about 4 minutes.
7. Remove the skillet from the heat and stir in the squash strands, sunflower seeds, and lemon juice.
8. Season with salt and pepper and serve warm.

Per Serving:calories: 218 / fat: 10g / protein: 5g / carbs: 32g / sugars: 13g / fiber: 7g / sodium: 232mg

Coconut Curry Rice

Prep time: 5 minutes / Cook time: 45 minutes / Serves 3

- 1 cup uncooked brown rice or brown basmati rice
- 1⅓ cups water
- 1 small can (5. 5 ounces) light coconut milk
- 2 tablespoons freshly squeezed lime juice
- 1 teaspoon mild curry powder
- Rounded ¼ teaspoon sea salt
- ¼ teaspoon turmeric powder
- 3–4 tablespoons chopped cilantro for serving (optional)
- Lime wedges for serving

1. In a saucepan, combine the rice, water, coconut milk, lime juice, curry powder, salt, and turmeric. Bring to a boil over high heat, stir, then reduce the heat to low. Cover and cook for 35 to 45 minutes, until the liquid is absorbed and the rice is tender.

Turn off the heat and let the rice sit, covered, for 5 minutes. Stir in the cilantro (if using), and serve with the lime wedges.

Per Serving:calorie: 298 / fat: 6g / protein: 6g / carbs: 56g / sugars: 2g / fiber: 4g / sodium: 303mg

Balsamic Green Beans and Fennel

Prep time: 20 minutes / Cook time: 18 minutes / Serves 4

- 2 teaspoons olive or canola oil
- 1 medium bulb fennel, cut into thin wedges
- 1 small onion, cut into thin wedges
- 2 cups frozen whole green beans
- ¼ cup water   • 2 teaspoons packed brown sugar
- ¼ teaspoon salt • ¼ teaspoon freshly ground pepper
- 1 tablespoon balsamic vinegar

1. In 12-inch nonstick skillet, heat oil over medium heat. Add fennel and onion; cook 7 to 8 minutes, stirring frequently, until fennel is light golden brown.
2. Add beans and water; heat to boiling. Stir; reduce heat to low. Cover; simmer 6 to 8 minutes or until beans are crisp-tender.
3. Stir in remaining ingredients; cook and stir 15 to 30 seconds longer or until vegetables are coated.

Per Serving:calorie: 80 / fat: 3g / protein: 1g / carbs: 13g / sugars: 6g / fiber: 4g / sodium: 180mg

Fennel and Chickpeas

Prep time: 10 minutes / Cook time: 20 minutes / Serves 6

- 1 tablespoon extra-virgin olive oil
- 1 small fennel bulb, trimmed and cut into ¼-inch-thick slices
- 1 sweet onion, thinly sliced
- 1 (15½-ounce) can sodium-free chickpeas, rinsed and drained
- 1 cup low-sodium chicken broth
- 2 teaspoons chopped fresh thyme
- ¼ teaspoon sea salt
- ¼ teaspoon freshly ground black pepper
- 1 tablespoon butter

1. Place a large saucepan over medium-high heat and add the oil.
2. Sauté the fennel and onion until tender and lightly browned, about 10 minutes.
3. Add the chickpeas, broth, thyme, salt, and pepper.
4. Cover and cook, stirring occasionally, for 10 minutes, until the liquid has reduced by about half.
5. Remove the pan from the heat and stir in the butter.
6. Serve hot.

Per Serving:calories: 132 / fat: 6g / protein:5 g / carbs: 17g / sugars: 6g / fiber: 4g / sodium: 239mg

Carrots Marsala

Prep time: 5 minutes / Cook time: 10 minutes / Serves 6

- 10 carrots (about 1 pound), peeled and diagonally sliced
- ¼ cup Marsala wine   • ¼ cup water
- 1 tablespoon extra-virgin olive oil
- ⅛ teaspoon freshly ground black pepper
- 1 tablespoon finely chopped fresh parsley

1. In a large saucepan, combine the carrots, wine, water, oil, and pepper. Bring to a boil, cover, reduce the heat, and simmer for 8 to 10 minutes, until the carrots are just tender, basting occasionally. Taste, and add salt, if desired.
2. Transfer to a serving dish, spoon any juices on top, and sprinkle with parsley.

Per Serving:calories: 48 / fat: 2g / protein: 1g / carbs: 6g / sugars: 3g / fiber: 2g / sodium: 46mg

Green Beans with Red Peppers

Prep time: 5 minutes / Cook time: 15 minutes / Serves 2

- 8 ounces fresh green beans, broken into 2-inch pieces
- 6 sun-dried tomatoes (not packed in oil), halved
- 1 medium red bell pepper, cut into ¼-inch strips
- 1 teaspoon extra-virgin olive oil
- Salt, to season
- Freshly ground black pepper, to season

1. In a 1-quart saucepan set over high heat, add the green beans to 1 inch of water. Bring to a boil. Boil for 5 minutes, uncovered.
2. Add the sun-dried tomatoes. Cover and boil 5 to 7 minutes more, or until the beans are crisp-tender, and the tomatoes have softened. Drain. Transfer to a serving bowl.
3. Add the red bell pepper and olive oil. Season with salt and pepper. Toss to coat.
4. Serve warm.

Per Serving:calories: 82 / fat: 3g / protein: 3g / carbs: 13g / sugars: 6g / fiber: 4g / sodium: 601mg

Sun-Dried Tomato Brussels Sprouts

Prep time: 15 minutes / Cook time: 20 minutes / Serves 4

- 1 pound Brussels sprouts, trimmed and halved
- 1 tablespoon extra-virgin olive oil
- Sea salt
- Freshly ground black pepper
- ½ cup sun-dried tomatoes, chopped
- 2 tablespoons freshly squeezed lemon juice
- 1 teaspoon lemon zest

1. Preheat the oven to 400°F. Line a large baking sheet with aluminum foil.
2. In a large bowl, toss the Brussels sprouts with oil and season with salt and pepper.
3. Spread the Brussels sprouts on the baking sheet in a single layer.
4. Roast the sprouts until they are caramelized, about

20 minutes.
5. Transfer the sprouts to a serving bowl. Mix in the sun-dried tomatoes, lemon juice, and lemon zest.
6. Stir to combine, and serve.

Per Serving:calories: 98 / fat: 4g / protein: 5g / carbs: 15g / sugars: 5g / fiber: 5g / sodium: 191mg

Best Brown Rice

Prep time: 5 minutes / Cook time: 22 minutes / Serves 6 to 12

- 2 cups brown rice
- 2½ cups water

1. Rinse brown rice in a fine-mesh strainer.
2. Add rice and water to the inner pot of the Instant Pot.
3. Secure the lid and make sure vent is on sealing.
4. Use Manual setting and select 22 minutes cooking time on high pressure.
5. When cooking time is done, let the pressure release naturally for 10 minutes, then press Cancel and manually release any remaining pressure.

Per Serving:calorie: 114 / fat: 1g / protein: 2g / carbs: 23g / sugars: 0g / fiber: 1g / sodium: 3mg

Artichokes Parmesan

Prep time: 5 minutes / Cook time: 20 minutes / Serves 6

- ½ cup dried whole-wheat bread crumbs
- 2 tablespoons grated Parmigiano-Reggiano cheese
- ⅛ teaspoon freshly ground black pepper
- 9 ounces frozen artichoke hearts, thawed
- 2 tablespoons extra-virgin olive oil, divided
- 2 medium tomatoes, diced

1. Preheat the oven to 425 degrees.
2. In a small bowl, combine the bread crumbs, cheese, and black pepper, and stir to combine.
3. Arrange the artichoke hearts in a 1-quart casserole dish. Sprinkle the tomatoes over the top. Season with salt, if desired.
4. Sprinkle the bread crumb mixture over the vegetables, and bake for 15–20 minutes or until the topping is light brown.

Per Serving:calories: 78 / fat: 5g / protein: 2g / carbs:7 g / sugars: 1g / fiber: 2g / sodium: 67mg

Callaloo Redux

Prep time: 15 minutes / Cook time: 25 minutes / Serves 6

- 3 cups store-bought low-sodium vegetable broth
- 1 (13½ ounces) can light coconut milk
- ¼ cup coconut cream
- 1 tablespoon unsalted non-hydrogenated plant-based butter
- 12 ounces okra, cut into 1-inch chunks
- 1 small onion, chopped
- ½ butternut squash, peeled, seeded, and cut into

4-inch chunks
- 1 bunch collard greens, stemmed and chopped
- 1 hot pepper (Scotch bonnet or habanero)

1. In an electric pressure cooker, combine the vegetable broth, coconut milk, coconut cream, and butter.
2. Layer the okra, onion, squash, collard greens, and whole hot pepper on top.
3. Close and lock the lid, and set the pressure valve to sealing.
4. Select the Manual/Pressure Cook setting, and cook for 20 minutes.
5. Once cooking is complete, quick-release the pressure. Carefully remove the lid.
6. Remove and discard the hot pepper. Carefully transfer the callaloo to a blender, and blend until smooth. Serve spooned over grits.

Per Serving:calories: 258 / fat: 21g / protein: 5g / carbs: 17g / sugars: 8g / fiber: 5g / sodium: 88mg

Not Slow-Cooked Collards

Prep time: 10 minutes / Cook time: 20 minutes / Serves 4

- 1 cup store-bought low-sodium vegetable broth, divided
- ½ onion, thinly sliced
- 2 garlic cloves, thinly sliced
- 1 large bunch collard greens including stems, roughly chopped
- 1 medium tomato, chopped
- 1 teaspoon ground cumin
- ½ teaspoon freshly ground black pepper

1. In a Dutch oven, bring ½ cup of broth to a simmer over medium heat.
2. Add the onion and garlic and cook for 3 to 5 minutes, or until translucent.
3. Add the collard greens, tomato, cumin, pepper, and the remaining ½ cup of broth, and gently stir.
4. Reduce the heat to low and cook, uncovered, for 15 minutes.

Per Serving:calories: 27 / fat: 0g / protein: 1g / carbs: 5g / sugars: 3g / fiber: 1g / sodium: 53mg

Roasted Eggplant

Prep time: 15 minutes / Cook time: 15 minutes / Serves 4

- 1 large eggplant
- 2 tablespoons olive oil
- ¼ teaspoon salt
- ½ teaspoon garlic powder

1. Remove top and bottom from eggplant. Slice eggplant into ¼-inch-thick round slices.
2. Brush slices with olive oil. Sprinkle with salt and garlic powder. Place eggplant slices into the air fryer basket.
3. Adjust the temperature to 390°F (199°C) and set the timer for 15 minutes.
4. Serve immediately.

Per Serving:calories: 98 / fat: 7g / protein: 2g / carbs: 8g / sugars: 3g / fiber: 3g / sodium: 200mg

Peas with Mushrooms and Thyme

Prep time: 10 minutes / Cook time: 10 minutes / Serves 6

- 2 teaspoons olive, canola or soybean oil
- 1 medium onion, diced (½ cup)
- 1 cup sliced fresh mushrooms
- 1 bag (16 ounces) frozen sweet peas
- ¼ teaspoon coarse (kosher or sea) salt
- ⅛ teaspoon white pepper
- 1 teaspoon chopped fresh or ¼ teaspoon dried thyme leaves

1. In 10-inch skillet, heat oil over medium heat. Add onion and mushrooms; cook 3 minutes, stirring occasionally. Stir in peas. Cook 3 to 5 minutes, stirring occasionally, until vegetables are tender.
2. Sprinkle with salt, pepper and thyme. Serve immediately.

Per Serving:calorie: 80 / fat: 1g / protein: 4g / carbs: 11g / sugars: 4g / fiber: 2g / sodium: 150mg

Asparagus-Pepper Stir-Fry

Prep time: 25 minutes / Cook time: 5 minutes / Serves 4

- 1 pound fresh asparagus spears
- 1 teaspoon canola oil
- 1 medium red, yellow or orange bell pepper, cut into ¾-inch pieces
- 2 cloves garlic, finely chopped
- 1 tablespoon orange juice
- 1 tablespoon reduced-sodium soy sauce
- ½ teaspoon ground ginger

1. Break off tough ends of asparagus as far down as stalks snap easily. Cut into 1-inch pieces.
2. In 10-inch nonstick skillet or wok, heat oil over medium heat. Add asparagus, bell pepper and garlic; cook 3 to 4 minutes or until crisp-tender, stirring constantly.
3. In small bowl, mix orange juice, soy sauce and ginger until blended; stir into asparagus mixture. Cook and stir 15 to 30 seconds or until vegetables are coated.

Per Serving:calorie: 40 / fat: 1. 5g / protein: 2g / carbs: 6g / sugars: 3g / fiber: 2g / sodium: 135mg

Chapter 8 Vegetarian Mains

Gingered Tofu and Greens

Prep time: 15 minutes / Cook time: 20 minutes / Serves 2

- For the marinade
- 2 tablespoons low-sodium soy sauce
- ¼ cup rice vinegar
- ⅓ cup water
- 1 tablespoon grated fresh ginger
- 1 tablespoon coconut flour
- 1 teaspoon granulated stevia
- 1 garlic clove, minced
- For the tofu and greens
- 8 ounces extra-firm tofu, drained, cut into 1-inch cubes
- 3 teaspoons extra-virgin olive oil, divided
- 1 tablespoon grated fresh ginger
- 2 cups coarsely shredded bok choy
- 2 cups coarsely shredded kale, thoroughly washed
- ½ cup fresh, or frozen, chopped green beans
- 1 tablespoon freshly squeezed lime juice
- 1 tablespoon chopped fresh cilantro
- 2 tablespoons hemp hearts

To make the marinade 1. In a small bowl, whisk together the soy sauce, rice vinegar, water, ginger, coconut flour, stevia, and garlic until well combined.

2. Place a small saucepan set over high heat. Add the marinade. Bring to a boil. Cook for 1 minute. Remove from the heat.

To make the tofu and greens 1. In a medium ovenproof pan, place the tofu in a single layer. Pour the marinade over. Drizzle with 1½ teaspoons of olive oil. Let sit for 5 minutes.

2. Preheat the broiler to high.

3. Place the pan under the broiler. Broil the tofu for 7 to 8 minutes, or until lightly browned. Using a spatula, turn the tofu over. Continue to broil for 7 to 8 minutes more, or until browned on this side.

4. In a large wok or skillet set over high heat, heat the remaining 1½ teaspoons of olive oil.

5. Stir in the ginger.

6. Add the bok choy, kale, and green beans. Cook for 2 to 3 minutes, stirring constantly, until the greens wilt.

7. Add the lime juice and cilantro. Remove from the heat.

8. Add the browned tofu with any remaining marinade in the pan to the bok choy, kale, and green beans. Toss gently to combine.

9. Top with the hemp hearts and serve immediately.

Per Serving: calories: 252 / fat: 14g / protein: 15g / carbs: 20g / sugars: 4g / fiber: 3g / sodium: 679mg

Stuffed Portobello Mushrooms

Prep time: 5 minutes / Cook time: 20 minutes / Serves 4

- 8 large portobello mushrooms
- 3 teaspoons extra-virgin olive oil, divided
- 4 cups fresh spinach
- 1 medium red bell pepper, diced
- ¼ cup crumbled feta

1. Preheat the oven to 450ºF.

2. Remove the stems from the mushrooms, and gently scoop out the gills and discard. Coat the mushrooms with 2 teaspoons of olive oil.

3. On a baking sheet, place the mushrooms cap-side down, and roast for 20 minutes.

4. Meanwhile, heat the remaining 1 teaspoon of olive oil in a medium skillet over medium heat. When hot, sauté the spinach and red bell pepper for 8 to 10 minutes, stirring occasionally.

5. Remove the mushrooms from the oven. Drain, if necessary. Spoon the spinach and pepper mix into the mushrooms, and top with feta.

Per Serving: calories: 91 / fat: 4g / protein: 6g / carbs: 10g / sugars: 3g / fiber: 4g / sodium: 155mg

Veggie Fajitas

Prep time: 10 minutes / Cook time: 15 minutes / Serves 4

- For The Guacamole
- 2 small avocados pitted and peeled
- 1 teaspoon freshly squeezed lime juice
- ¼ teaspoon salt
- 9 cherry tomatoes, halved
- For The Fajitas
- 1 red bell pepper
- 1 green bell pepper
- 1 small white onion
- Avocado oil cooking spray
- 1 cup canned low-sodium black beans, drained and rinsed
- ½ teaspoon ground cumin
- ¼ teaspoon chili powder
- ¼ teaspoon garlic powder
- 4 (6-inch) yellow corn tortillas

To Make The Guacamole 1. In a medium bowl, use a fork to mash the avocados with the lime juice and salt.

2. Gently stir in the cherry tomatoes.

To Make The Fajitas 1. Cut the red bell pepper, green bell pepper, and onion into ½-inch slices.

2. Heat a large skillet over medium heat. When hot,

coat the cooking surface with cooking spray. Put the peppers, onion, and beans into the skillet.

3. Add the cumin, chili powder, and garlic powder, and stir.
4. Cover and cook for 15 minutes, stirring halfway through.
5. Divide the fajita mixture equally between the tortillas, and top with guacamole and any preferred garnishes.

Per Serving:calories: 269 / fat: 15g / protein: 8g / carbs: 30g / sugars: 5g / fiber: 11g / sodium: 175mg

Chickpea and Tofu Bolognese

Prep time: 5 minutes / Cook time: 25 minutes / Serves 4

- 1 (3 to 4 pounds) spaghetti squash
- ½ teaspoon ground cumin
- 1 cup no-sugar-added spaghetti sauce
- 1 (15 ounces) can low-sodium chickpeas, drained and rinsed
- 6 ounces extra-firm tofu

1. Preheat the oven to 400ºF.
2. Cut the squash in half lengthwise. Scoop out the seeds and discard.
3. Season both halves of the squash with the cumin, and place them on a baking sheet cut-side down. Roast for 25 minutes.
4. Meanwhile, heat a medium saucepan over low heat, and pour in the spaghetti sauce and chickpeas.
5. Press the tofu between two layers of paper towels, and gently squeeze out any excess water.
6. Crumble the tofu into the sauce and cook for 15 minutes.
7. Remove the squash from the oven, and comb through the flesh of each half with a fork to make thin strands.
8. Divide the "spaghetti" into four portions, and top each portion with one-quarter of the sauce.

Per Serving:calories: 221 / fat: 6g / protein: 12g / carbs: 32g / sugars: 6g / fiber: 8g / sodium: 405mg

Edamame Falafel with Roasted Vegetables

Prep time: 10 minutes / Cook time: 55 minutes / Serves 2

- For the roasted vegetables
- 1 cup broccoli florets
- 1 medium zucchini, sliced
- ½ cup cherry tomatoes, halved
- 1½ teaspoons extra-virgin olive oil
- Salt, to season
- Freshly ground black pepper, to season
- Extra-virgin olive oil cooking spray
- For the falafel
- 1 cup frozen shelled edamame, thawed
- 1 small onion, chopped

- 1 garlic clove, chopped
- 1 tablespoon freshly squeezed lemon juice
- 2 tablespoons hemp hearts
- 1 teaspoon ground cumin
- 2 tablespoons oat flour
- ¼ teaspoon salt
- Pinch freshly ground black pepper
- 2 tablespoons extra-virgin olive oil, divided
- Prepared hummus, for serving (optional)

To make the roasted vegetables 1. Preheat the oven to 425°F.
2. In a large bowl, toss together the broccoli, zucchini, tomatoes, and olive oil to coat. Season with salt and pepper.
3. Spray a baking sheet with cooking spray.
4. Spread the vegetables evenly atop the sheet. Place the sheet in the preheated oven. Roast for 35 to 40 minutes, stirring every 15 minutes, or until the vegetables are soft and cooked through.
5. Remove from the oven. Set aside.

To make the falafel 1. In a food processor, pulse the edamame until coarsely ground.
2. Add the onion, garlic, lemon juice, and hemp hearts. Process until finely ground. Transfer the mixture to a medium bowl.
3. By hand, mix in the cumin, oat flour, salt, and pepper.
4. Roll the dough into 1-inch balls. Flatten slightly. You should have about 12 silver dollar–size patties.
5. In a large skillet set over medium heat, heat 1 tablespoon of olive oil.
6. Add 4 falafel patties to the pan at a time (or as many as will fit without crowding), and cook for about 3 minutes on each side, or until lightly browned. Remove from the pan. Repeat with the remaining 1 tablespoon of olive oil and falafel patties.
7. Serve immediately with the roasted vegetables and hummus (if using) and enjoy!

Per Serving:calories: 316 / fat: 22g / protein: 12g / carbs: 21g / sugars: 4g / fiber: 6g / sodium: 649mg

Southwest Tofu

Prep time: 10 minutes / Cook time: 20 minutes / Serves 4

- 3½ tablespoons freshly squeezed lime juice
- 2 teaspoons pure maple syrup
- 1½ teaspoons ground cumin
- 1 teaspoon dried oregano leaves
- 1 teaspoon chili powder
- ½ teaspoon paprika
- ½ teaspoon sea salt
- ⅛ teaspoon allspice
- 1 package (12 ounces) extra-firm tofu, sliced into ¼"–½" thick squares and patted to remove excess moisture

1. In a 9" x 12" baking dish, combine the lime juice, syrup, cumin, oregano, chili powder, paprika, salt, and allspice. Add the tofu and turn to coat both sides. Bake uncovered for 20 minutes, or until the marinade is absorbed, turning once.

Per Serving:calorie: 78 / fat: 4g / protein: 7g / carbs: 6g / sugars: 3g / fiber: 1g / sodium: 324mg

Italian Tofu with Mushrooms and Peppers

Prep time: 5 minutes / Cook time: 10 minutes / Serves 2

- 1 teaspoon extra-virgin olive oil
- ¼ cup chopped bell pepper, any color
- ¼ cup chopped onions
- 1 garlic clove, minced
- 8 ounces firm tofu, drained and rinsed
- ½ cup sliced fresh button mushrooms
- 1 portobello mushroom cap, chopped
- 1 tablespoon balsamic vinegar
- 1 teaspoon dried basil
- Salt, to season
- Freshly ground black pepper, to season

1. In a medium skillet set over medium heat, heat the olive oil.
2. Add the bell pepper, onions, and garlic. Sauté for 5 minutes, or until soft.
3. Add the tofu, button mushrooms, and portobello mushrooms, tossing and stirring. Reduce the heat to low.
4. Stir in the balsamic vinegar and basil. Season with salt and pepper. Simmer for 2 minutes.
5. Enjoy!

Per Serving:calories: 142 / fat: 8g / protein: 13g / carbs: 9g / sugars: 4g / fiber: 2g / sodium: 326mg

Crispy Cabbage Steaks

Prep time: 5 minutes / Cook time: 10 minutes / Serves 4

- 1 small head green cabbage, cored and cut into ½-inch-thick slices
- ¼ teaspoon salt
- ¼ teaspoon ground black pepper
- 2 tablespoons olive oil
- 1 clove garlic, peeled and finely minced
- ½ teaspoon dried thyme
- ½ teaspoon dried parsley

1. Sprinkle each side of cabbage with salt and pepper, then place into ungreased air fryer basket, working in batches if needed.
2. Drizzle each side of cabbage with olive oil, then sprinkle with remaining ingredients on both sides. Adjust the temperature to 350°F (177°C) and air fry for 10 minutes, turning "steaks" halfway through cooking. 3. Cabbage will be browned at the edges and tender when done. Serve warm.

Per Serving:calorie: 90 / fat: 7g / protein: 2g / carbs: 7g / sugars: 3g / fiber: 3g / sodium: 170mg

Easy Cheesy Vegetable Frittata

Prep time: 10 minutes / Cook time: 15 minutes / Serves 2

- Extra-virgin olive oil cooking spray
- ½ cup sliced onion
- ½ cup sliced green bell pepper
- ½ cup sliced eggplant
- ½ cup frozen spinach
- ½ cup sliced fresh mushrooms
- 1 tablespoon chopped fresh basil
- Pinch freshly ground black pepper
- ½ cup liquid egg substitute
- ½ cup nonfat cottage cheese
- ¼ cup fat-free evaporated milk
- ¼ cup nonfat shredded Cheddar cheese

1. Coat an ovenproof 10-inch skillet with cooking spray. Place it over medium-low heat until hot.
2. Add the onion, green bell pepper, eggplant, spinach, and mushrooms. Sauté for 2 to 3 minutes, or until lightly browned.
3. Add the basil. Season with pepper. Stir to combine. Cook for 2 to 3 minutes more, or until the flavors blend. Remove from the heat.
4. Preheat the broiler.
5. In a blender, combine the egg substitute, cottage cheese, Cheddar cheese, and evaporated milk. Process until smooth. Pour the egg mixture over the vegetables in the skillet.
6. Return the skillet to medium-low heat. Cover and cook for about 5 minutes, or until the bottom sets and the top is still slightly wet.
7. Transfer the ovenproof skillet to the broiler. Broil for 2 to 3 minutes, or until the top is set.
8. Serve one-half of the frittata per person and enjoy!

Per Serving:calories: 177 / fat: 7g / protein: 17g / carbs: 12g / sugars: 6g / fiber: 3g / sodium: 408mg

Mushroom and Cauliflower Rice Risotto

Prep time: 5 minutes / Cook time: 10 minutes / Serves 4

- 1 teaspoon extra-virgin olive oil
- ½ cup chopped portobello mushrooms
- 4 cups cauliflower rice
- ¼ cup low-sodium vegetable broth
- ½ cup half-and-half
- 1 cup shredded Parmesan cheese

1. Heat the oil in a medium skillet over medium-low heat. When hot, put the mushrooms in the skillet and cook for 3 minutes, stirring once.
2. Add the cauliflower rice, broth, and half-and-half. Stir and cover. Increase to high heat and boil for 5 minutes.

3. Add the cheese. Stir to incorporate. Cook for 3 more minutes.

Per Serving:calories: 159 / fat: 8g / protein: 10g / carbs: 12g / sugars: 4g / fiber: 2g / sodium: 531mg

Spinach Salad with Eggs, Tempeh Bacon, and Strawberries

Prep time: 10 minutes / Cook time: 15 minutes / Serves 4

- 2 tablespoons soy sauce, tamari, or coconut aminos
- 1 tablespoon raw apple cider vinegar
- 1 tablespoon pure maple syrup
- ½ teaspoon smoked paprika
- Freshly ground black pepper
- One 8-ounce package tempeh, cut crosswise into ⅛-inch-thick slices
- 8 large eggs
- 3 tablespoons extra-virgin olive oil
- 1 shallot, minced
- 1 tablespoon red wine vinegar
- 1 tablespoon balsamic vinegar
- 1 teaspoon Dijon mustard
- ¼ teaspoon fine sea salt
- One 6-ounce bag baby spinach
- 2 hearts romaine lettuce, torn into bite-size pieces
- 12 fresh strawberries, sliced

1. In a 1-quart ziplock plastic bag, combine the soy sauce, cider vinegar, maple syrup, paprika, and ½ teaspoon pepper and carefully agitate the bag to mix the ingredients to make a marinade. Add the tempeh, seal the bag, and turn the bag back and forth several times to coat the tempeh evenly with the marinade. Marinate in the refrigerator for at least 2 hours or up to 24 hours.
2. Pour 1 cup water into the Instant Pot and place the wire metal steam rack, an egg rack, or a steamer basket into the pot. Gently place the eggs on top of the rack or in the basket, taking care not to crack them.
3. Secure the lid and set the Pressure Release to Sealing. Select the Steam setting and set the cooking time for 3 minutes at high pressure. (The pot will take about 5 minutes to come up to pressure before the cooking program begins.)
4. While the eggs are cooking, prepare an ice bath.
5. When the cooking program ends, perform a quick pressure release by moving the Pressure Release to Venting. Open the pot and, using tongs, transfer the eggs to the ice bath to cool.
6. Remove the tempeh from the marinade and blot dry between layers of paper towels. Discard the marinade. In a large nonstick skillet over medium-high heat, warm 1 tablespoon of the oil for 2 minutes. Add the tempeh in a single layer and fry, turning once, for 2 to 3 minutes per side, until well

browned. Transfer the tempeh to a plate and set aside.
7. Wipe out the skillet and set it over medium heat. Add the remaining 2 tablespoons oil and the shallot and sauté for about 2 minutes, until the shallot is golden brown. Turn off the heat and stir in the red wine vinegar, balsamic vinegar, mustard, salt, and ¼ teaspoon pepper to make a vinaigrette.
8. In a large bowl, combine the spinach and romaine. Pour in the vinaigrette and toss until all of the leaves are lightly coated. Divide the dressed greens evenly among four large serving plates or shallow bowls and arrange the strawberries and fried tempeh on top. Peel the eggs, cut them in half lengthwise, and place them on top of the salads. Top with a couple grinds of pepper and serve right away.

Per Serving:calorie: 435 / fat: 25g / protein: 29g / carbs: 25g / sugars: 10g / fiber: 5g / sodium: 332mg

Chile Relleno Casserole with Salsa Salad

Prep time: 10 minutes / Cook time: 55 minutes / Serves 4

- Casserole
- ½ cup gluten-free flour (such as King Arthur)
- 1 teaspoon baking powder
- 6 large eggs
- ½ cup nondairy milk or whole milk
- Three 4 ounces cans fire-roasted diced green chiles, drained
- 1 cup nondairy cheese shreds or shredded mozzarella cheese
- Salad
- 1 head green leaf lettuce, shredded
- 2 Roma tomatoes, seeded and diced
- 1 green bell pepper, seeded and diced
- ½ small yellow onion, diced
- 1 jalapeño chile, seeded and diced (optional)
- 2 tablespoons chopped fresh cilantro
- 4 teaspoons extra-virgin olive oil
- 4 teaspoons fresh lime juice
- ⅛ teaspoon fine sea salt

1. To make the casserole: Pour 1 cup water into the Instant Pot. Butter a 7-cup round heatproof glass dish or coat with nonstick cooking spray and place the dish on a long-handled silicone steam rack. (If you don't have the long-handled rack, use the wire metal steam rack and a homemade sling)
2. In a medium bowl, whisk together the flour and baking powder. Add the eggs and milk and whisk until well blended, forming a batter. Stir in the chiles and ¾ cup of the cheese.
3. Pour the batter into the prepared dish and cover tightly with aluminum foil. Holding the handles of the steam rack, lower the dish into the Instant Pot.
4. Secure the lid and set the Pressure Release to

Sealing. Select the Pressure Cook or Manual setting and set the cooking time for 40 minutes at high pressure. (The pot will take about 10 minutes to come up to pressure before the cooking program begins.)

5. When the cooking program ends, let the pressure release naturally for at least 10 minutes, then move the Pressure Release to Venting to release any remaining steam. Open the pot and, wearing heat-resistant mitts, grasp the handles of the steam rack and lift it out of the pot. Uncover the dish, taking care not to get burned by the steam or to drip condensation onto the casserole. While the casserole is still piping hot, sprinkle the remaining ¼ cup cheese evenly on top. Let the cheese melt for 5 minutes.

6. To make the salad: While the cheese is melting, in a large bowl, combine the lettuce, tomatoes, bell pepper, onion, jalapeño (if using), cilantro, oil, lime juice, and salt. Toss until evenly combined.

7. Cut the casserole into wedges. Serve warm, with the salad on the side.

Per Serving:calorie: 361 / fat: 22g / protein: 21g / carbs: 23g / sugars: 8g / fiber: 3g / sodium: 421mg

Cheesy Zucchini Patties

Prep time: 10 minutes / Cook time: 20 minutes / Serves 2

- 1 cup grated zucchini
- 1 cup chopped fresh mushrooms
- ½ cup grated carrot
- ½ cup nonfat shredded mozzarella cheese
- ¼ cup finely ground flaxseed
- 1 large egg, beaten
- 1 garlic clove, minced
- Salt, to season
- Freshly ground black pepper, to season
- 1 tablespoon extra-virgin olive oil
- 4 cup mixed baby greens, divided

1. In a medium bowl, stir together the zucchini, mushrooms, carrot, mozzarella cheese, flaxseed, egg, and garlic. Season with salt and pepper. Stir again to combine.

2. In a large skillet set over medium-high heat, heat the olive oil.

3. Drop 1 tablespoon of the zucchini mixture into the skillet. Continue dropping tablespoon-size portions in the pan until it is full, but not crowded. Cook for 2 to 3 minutes on each side, or until golden. Transfer to a serving plate. Repeat with the remaining mixture.

4. Place 2 cups of greens on each serving plate. Top each with zucchini patties.

5. Enjoy!

Per Serving:calories: 252 / fat: 15g / protein: 19g / carbs:

14g / sugars: 4g / fiber: 9g / sodium: 644mg

Vegan Dal Makhani

Prep time: 0 minutes / Cook time: 55 minutes / Serves 6

- 1 cup dried kidney beans
- ⅓ cup urad dal or beluga or Puy lentils
- 4 cups water
- 1 teaspoon fine sea salt
- 1 tablespoon cold-pressed avocado oil
- 1 tablespoon cumin seeds
- 1-inch piece fresh ginger, peeled and minced
- 4 garlic cloves, minced
- 1 large yellow onion, diced
- 2 jalapeño chiles, seeded and diced
- 1 green bell pepper, seeded and diced
- 1 tablespoon garam masala
- 1 teaspoon ground turmeric
- ¼ teaspoon cayenne pepper (optional)
- One 15-ounce can fire-roasted diced tomatoes and liquid
- 2 tablespoons vegan buttery spread
- Cooked cauliflower "rice" for serving
- 2 tablespoons chopped fresh cilantro
- 6 tablespoons plain coconut yogurt

1. In a medium bowl, combine the kidney beans, urad dal, water, and salt and stir to dissolve the salt. Let soak for 12 hours.

2. Select the Sauté setting on the Instant Pot and heat the oil and cumin seeds for 3 minutes, until the seeds are bubbling, lightly toasted, and aromatic. Add the ginger and garlic and sauté for 1 minute, until bubbling and fragrant. Add the onion, jalapeños, and bell pepper and sauté for 5 minutes, until the onion begins to soften.

3. Add the garam masala, turmeric, cayenne (if using), and the soaked beans and their liquid and stir to mix. Pour the tomatoes and their liquid on top. Do not stir them in.

4. Secure the lid and set the Pressure Release to Sealing. Press the Cancel button to reset the cooking program, then select the Pressure Cook or Manual setting and set the cooking time for 30 minutes at high pressure. (The pot will take about 15 minutes to come up to pressure before the cooking program begins.)

5. When the cooking program ends, let the pressure release naturally for 30 minutes, then move the Pressure Release to Venting to release any remaining steam. Open the pot and stir to combine, then stir in the buttery spread. If you prefer a smoother texture, ladle 1½ cups of the dal into a blender and blend until smooth, about 30 seconds, then stir the blended mixture into the rest of the dal in the pot.

6. Spoon the cauliflower "rice" into bowls and ladle the dal on top. Sprinkle with the cilantro, top with a dollop of coconut yogurt, and serve.

Per Serving:calorie: 245 / fat: 7g / protein: 11g / carbs: 37g / sugars: 4g / fiber: 10g / sodium: 518mg

Greek Stuffed Eggplant

Prep time: 15 minutes / Cook time: 20 minutes / Serves 2

- 1 large eggplant
- 2 tablespoons unsalted butter
- ¼ medium yellow onion, diced
- ¼ cup chopped artichoke hearts
- 1 cup fresh spinach
- 2 tablespoons diced red bell pepper
- ½ cup crumbled feta

1. Slice eggplant in half lengthwise and scoop out flesh, leaving enough inside for shell to remain intact. Take eggplant that was scooped out, chop it, and set aside.
2. In a medium skillet over medium heat, add butter and onion. Sauté until onions begin to soften, about 3 to 5 minutes. Add chopped eggplant, artichokes, spinach, and bell pepper. Continue cooking 5 minutes until peppers soften and spinach wilts. Remove from the heat and gently fold in the feta.
3. Place filling into each eggplant shell and place into the air fryer basket.
4. Adjust the temperature to 320ºF (160ºC) and air fry for 20 minutes.
5. Eggplant will be tender when done. Serve warm.

Per Serving:calories: 259 / fat: 16g / protein: 10g / carbs: 22g / sugars: 12g / fiber: 10g / sodium: 386mg

Black-Eyed Pea Sauté with Garlic and Olives

Prep time: 5 minutes / Cook time: 5 minutes / Serves 2

- 2 teaspoons extra-virgin olive oil
- 1 garlic clove, minced
- ½ red onion, chopped
- 1 cup cooked black-eyed peas; if canned, drain and rinse
- ½ teaspoon dried thyme
- ¼ cup water
- ¼ teaspoon salt
- ¼ teaspoon freshly ground black pepper
- 6 Kalamata olives, pitted and halved

1. In a medium saucepan set over medium heat, stir together the olive oil, garlic, and red onion. Cook for 2 minutes, continuing to stir.
2. Add the black-eyed peas and thyme. Cook for 1 minute.
3. Stir in the water, salt, pepper, and olives. Cook for 2 minutes more, or until heated through.

Per Serving:calories: 140 / fat: 6g / protein: 5g / carbs: 18g / sugars: 8g / fiber: 5g / sodium: 426mg

Italian Zucchini Boats

Prep time: 5 minutes / Cook time: 15 minutes / Serves 4

- 1 cup canned low-sodium chickpeas, drained and rinsed
- 1 cup no-sugar-added spaghetti sauce
- 2 zucchini
- ¼ cup shredded Parmesan cheese

1. Preheat the oven to 425ºF.
2. In a medium bowl, mix the chickpeas and spaghetti sauce together.
3. Cut the zucchini in half lengthwise, and scrape a spoon gently down the length of each half to remove the seeds.
4. Fill each zucchini half with the chickpea sauce, and top with one-quarter of the Parmesan cheese.
5. Place the zucchini halves on a baking sheet and roast in the oven for 15 minutes.

Per Serving:calories: 120 / fat: 4g / protein: 7g / carbs: 14g / sugars: 5g / fiber: 4g / sodium: 441mg

Chickpea Coconut Curry

Prep time: 5 minutes / Cook time: 15 minutes / Serves 4

- 3 cups fresh or frozen cauliflower florets
- 2 cups unsweetened almond milk
- 1 (15 ounces) can coconut milk
- 1 (15 ounces) can low-sodium chickpeas, drained and rinsed
- 1 tablespoon curry powder
- ¼ teaspoon ground ginger
- ¼ teaspoon garlic powder
- ⅛ teaspoon onion powder
- ¼ teaspoon salt

1. In a large stockpot, combine the cauliflower, almond milk, coconut milk, chickpeas, curry, ginger, garlic powder, and onion powder. Stir and cover.
2. Cook over medium-high heat for 10 minutes.
3. Reduce the heat to low, stir, and cook for 5 minutes more, uncovered. Season with up to ¼ teaspoon salt.

Per Serving:calories: 225 / fat: 7g / protein: 12g / carbs: 31g / sugars: 14g / fiber: 9g / sodium: 489mg

Caprese Eggplant Stacks

Prep time: 5 minutes / Cook time: 12 minutes / Serves 4

- 1 medium eggplant, cut into ¼-inch slices
- 2 large tomatoes, cut into ¼-inch slices
- 4 ounces (113 g) fresh Mozzarella, cut into ½-ounce / 14-g slices
- 2 tablespoons olive oil
- ¼ cup fresh basil, sliced

1. In a baking dish, place four slices of eggplant on

the bottom. Place a slice of tomato on top of each eggplant round, then Mozzarella, then eggplant. Repeat as necessary.
2. Drizzle with olive oil. Cover dish with foil and place dish into the air fryer basket.
3. Adjust the temperature to 350°F (177°C) and bake for 12 minutes.
4. When done, eggplant will be tender. Garnish with fresh basil to serve.

Per Serving:calories: 216 / fat: 16g / protein: 9g / carbs: 11g / sugars: 6g / fiber: 5g / sodium: 231mg

Vegetable Burgers

Prep time: 10 minutes / Cook time: 12 minutes / Serves 4

- 8 ounces (227 g) cremini mushrooms
- 2 large egg yolks
- ½ medium zucchini, trimmed and chopped
- ¼ cup peeled and chopped yellow onion
- 1 clove garlic, peeled and finely minced
- ½ teaspoon salt
- ¼ teaspoon ground black pepper

1. Place all ingredients into a food processor and pulse twenty times until finely chopped and combined.
2. Separate mixture into four equal sections and press each into a burger shape. Place burgers into ungreased air fryer basket. Adjust the temperature to 375°F (191°C) and air fry for 12 minutes, turning burgers halfway through cooking. Burgers will be browned and firm when done.
3. Place burgers on a large plate and let cool 5 minutes before serving.

Per Serving:calories: 77 / fat: 5g / protein: 3g / carbs: 6g / sugars: 2g / fiber: 1g / sodium: 309mg

Chickpea-Spinach Curry

Prep time: 5 minutes / Cook time: 10 minutes / Serves 2

- 1 cup frozen chopped spinach, thawed
- 1 cup canned chickpeas, drained and rinsed
- ½ cup frozen green beans
- ½ cup frozen broccoli florets
- ½ cup no-salt-added canned chopped tomatoes, undrained
- 1 tablespoon curry powder
- 1 tablespoon granulated garlic
- Salt, to season
- Freshly ground black pepper, to season
- ½ cup chopped fresh parsley

1. In a medium saucepan set over high heat, stir together the spinach, chickpeas, green beans, broccoli, tomatoes and their juice, curry powder, and garlic. Season with salt and pepper. Bring to a fast boil. Reduce the heat to low. Cover and simmer for 10 minutes, or until heated through.

2. Top with the parsley, serve, and enjoy!

Per Serving:calories: 203 / fat: 3g / protein: 13g / carbs: 35g / sugars: 7g / fiber: 13g / sodium: 375mg

Grilled Vegetables on White Bean Mash

Prep time: 15 minutes / Cook time: 30 minutes / Serves 2

- 2 medium zucchini, sliced
- 1 red bell pepper, seeded and quartered
- 2 portobello mushroom caps, quartered
- 3 teaspoons extra-virgin olive oil, divided
- 1 (8-ounce) can cannellini beans, drained and rinsed
- 1 garlic clove, minced
- ½ cup low-sodium vegetable broth
- 4 cups baby spinach, divided
- Salt, to season
- Freshly ground black pepper, to season
- 1 tablespoon chopped fresh parsley
- 2 lemon wedges, divided, for garnish

1. Preheat the grill. Use a stove-top grill pan or broiler if a grill is not available.
2. Lightly brush the zucchini, red bell pepper, and mushrooms with 1½ teaspoons of olive oil. Arrange them in a barbecue grill pan. Place the pan on the preheated grill. Cook the vegetables for 5 to 8 minutes, or until lightly browned. Turn the vegetables. Brush with the remaining 1½ teaspoons of olive oil. Cook for 5 to 8 minutes more, or until tender.
3. To a small pan set over high heat, add the cannellini beans, garlic, and vegetable broth. Bring to a boil. Reduce the heat to low. Simmer for 10 minutes, uncovered. Using a potato masher, roughly mash the beans, adding a little more broth if they seem too dry.
4. Place 2 cups of spinach on each serving plate.
5. Top each with half of the bean mash and half of the grilled vegetables. Season with salt and pepper. Garnish with parsley.
6. Place 1 lemon wedge on each plate and serve.

Per Serving:calories: 290 / fat: 9g / protein: 11g / carbs:29 g / sugars: 8g / fiber: 4g / sodium: 398mg

Pra Ram Vegetables and Peanut Sauce with Seared Tofu

Prep time: 5 minutes / Cook time: 20 minutes / Serves 4

- Peanut Sauce
- 2 tablespoons cold-pressed avocado oil
- 2 garlic cloves, minced
- ½ cup creamy natural peanut butter
- ½ cup coconut milk
- 2 tablespoons brown rice syrup
- 1 tablespoon plus 1 teaspoon soy sauce, tamari, or coconut aminos

- ¼ cup water
- Vegetables
- 2 carrots, sliced on the diagonal ¼ inch thick
- 8 ounces zucchini, julienned ¼ inch thick
- 1 pound broccoli florets
- ½ small head green cabbage, cut into 1-inch-thick wedges (with core intact so wedges hold together)
- Tofu
- One 14-ounce package extra-firm tofu, drained
- ¼ teaspoon fine sea salt
- ¼ teaspoon freshly ground black pepper
- 1 tablespoon cornstarch
- 2 tablespoons coconut oil

1. To make the peanut sauce: In a small saucepan over medium heat, warm the oil and garlic for about 2 minutes, until the garlic is bubbling but not browned. Add the peanut butter, coconut milk, brown rice syrup, soy sauce, and water; stir to combine; and bring to a simmer (this will take about 3 minutes). As soon as the mixture is fully combined and at a simmer, remove from the heat and keep warm. The peanut sauce will keep in an airtight container in the refrigerator for up to 5 days.
2. To make the vegetables: Pour 1 cup water into the Instant Pot and place a steamer basket into the pot. In order, layer the carrots, zucchini, broccoli, and cabbage in the steamer basket, finishing with the cabbage.
3. Secure the lid and set the Pressure Release to Sealing. Select the Steam setting and set the cooking time for 0 (zero) minutes at low pressure. (The pot will take about 15 minutes to come up to pressure before the cooking program begins.)
4. To prepare the tofu: While the vegetables are steaming, cut the tofu crosswise into eight ½-inch-thick slices. Cut each of the slices in half crosswise, creating squares. Sandwich the squares between double layers of paper towels or a folded kitchen towel and press firmly to wick away as much moisture as possible. Sprinkle the tofu squares on both sides with the salt and pepper, then sprinkle them on both sides with the cornstarch. Using your fingers, spread the cornstarch on the top and bottom of each square to coat evenly.
5. In a large nonstick skillet over medium-high heat, warm the oil for about 3 minutes, until shimmering. Add the tofu and sear, turning once, for about 6 minutes per side, until crispy and golden. Divide the tofu evenly among four plates.
6. When the cooking program ends, perform a quick pressure release by moving the Pressure Release to

Venting. Open the pot and, wearing heat-resistant mitts, grasp the handles of the steamer basket and lift it out of the pot.
7. Divide the vegetables among the plates, arranging them around the tofu. Spoon the peanut sauce over the tofu and serve.

Per Serving:calories: 380 / fat: 22g / protein: 18g / carbs: 30g / sugars: 9g / fiber: 10g / sodium: 381mg

Quinoa–White Bean Loaf

Prep time: 15 minutes / Cook time: 1 hour / Serves 2

- Extra-virgin olive oil cooking spray
- 2 teaspoons extra-virgin olive oil
- 2 garlic cloves, minced
- ½ cup sliced fresh button mushrooms
- 6 ounces extra-firm tofu, crumbled
- Salt, to season
- Freshly ground black pepper, to season
- 1 (8-ounce) can cannellini beans, drained and rinsed
- 2 tablespoons coconut flour
- 1 tablespoon chia seeds
- ⅓ cup water
- ½ cup cooked quinoa
- ¼ cup chopped red onion
- ¼ cup chopped fresh parsley

1. Preheat the oven to 350°F.
2. Lightly coat 2 mini loaf pans with cooking spray. Set aside.
3. In a large skillet set over medium-high heat, heat the olive oil.
4. Add the garlic, mushrooms, and tofu. Season with salt and pepper.
5. Cook for 6 to 8 minutes, stirring occasionally, until the mushrooms and tofu are golden brown.
6. In a food processor, combine the cannellini beans, coconut flour, chia seeds, and water. Pulse until almost smooth.
7. In a large bowl, mix together the mushroom and tofu mixture, cannellini bean mixture, quinoa, red onion, and parsley. Season with salt and pepper.
8. Evenly divide the mixture between the 2 prepared loaf pans, gently pressing down and mounding the mixture in the middle.
9. Place the pans in the preheated oven. Bake for about 1 hour, or until firm and golden brown. Remove from the oven. Let rest for 10 minutes.
10. Slice and serve.

Per Serving:calories: 193 / fat: 8g / protein: 12g / carbs: 20g / sugars: 4g / fiber: 4g / sodium: 366mg

Chapter 9 Desserts

Classic Crêpes

Prep time: 30 minutes / Cook time: 10 minutes / Serves 10

- ¾ cup egg substitute
- 1⅓ cups buckwheat flour
- ½ teaspoon salt
- 1½ cups fat-free milk
- 2 teaspoons canola oil

1. In a food processor or blender, combine all ingredients. Process for 30 seconds, scraping down the sides of the container. Continue to process until the mixture is smooth; refrigerate for 1 hour.
2. Coat the bottom of a 6-inch crêpe pan or small skillet with nonstick cooking spray. Place the pan over medium heat until hot but not smoking.
3. Pour 2 tablespoons of the batter into the pan, and quickly tilt it in all directions so the batter covers the pan in a thin film. Cook for about 1 minute, lifting the edge of the crêpe to test for doneness. The crêpe is ready to be flipped when it can be shaken loose from the pan.
4. Flip the crêpe, and continue to cook for 30 seconds on the other side. (This side usually has brownish spots on it, so place the filling on this side.)
5. Stack the cooked crêpes between layers of wax paper to avoid sticking, and repeat the process with the remaining batter.

Per Serving:calories: 83 / fat: 1g / protein: 5g / carbs: 13g / sugars: 3g / fiber: 2g / sodium: 173mg

Dulce de Leche Fillo Cups

Prep time: 15 minutes / Cook time: 0 minutes / Serves 15

- 2 ounces ⅓-less-fat cream cheese (Neufchâtel), softened
- 2 tablespoons dulce de leche (caramel) syrup
- 1 tablespoon reduced-fat sour cream
- 1 package frozen mini fillo shells (15 shells)
- ⅓ cup sliced fresh strawberries
- 2 tablespoons diced mango

1. In medium bowl, beat cream cheese with electric mixer on low speed until creamy. Beat in dulce de leche syrup and sour cream until blended.
2. Spoon cream cheese mixture into each fillo shell. Top each with strawberries and mango.

Per Serving:calorie: 40 / fat: 2g / protein: 0g / carbs: 4g / sugars: 2g / fiber: 0g / sodium: 35mg

No-Added-Sugar Orange and Cream Slushy

Prep time: 5 minutes / Cook time: 0 minutes / Serves 2

- ½ cup (120 ml) unsweetened vanilla almond milk
- ½ cup (100 g) plain whole-milk yogurt
- 2 small oranges, peeled, seeds and pith removed, and frozen
- 1 small banana, frozen
- 1 teaspoon pure vanilla extract
- 2 tablespoons (10 g) unsweetened coconut flakes
- 1 tablespoon (12 g) chia seeds

1. In a high-power blender, combine the almond milk, yogurt, oranges, banana, vanilla, coconut flakes, and chia seeds. Blend the ingredients for 30 to 45 seconds, until a slushy consistency is reached.

Per Serving:calorie: 203 / fat: 7g / protein: 8g / carbs: 29g / sugars: 17g / fiber: 7g / sodium: 67mg

Banana N'Ice Cream with Cocoa Nuts

Prep time: 10 minutes / Cook time: 12 minutes / Serves 4 to 6

- For the Cocoa Nuts:
- ¼ cup freshly squeezed orange juice
- 1 tablespoon coconut oil
- 2 teaspoons cocoa powder
- ½ teaspoon kosher salt
- ¼ teaspoon ground cinnamon
- ¼ teaspoon ground cardamom
- ½ teaspoon orange zest
- 1 cup raw almonds
- For the Banana N'ice Cream:
- 2 frozen, diced bananas

Make the Cocoa Nuts: 1. Preheat the oven to 350°F. Line a baking sheet with parchment paper.
2. In a small saucepan, bring the orange juice to a boil over medium-high heat, reduce the heat to low, and simmer until the juice is reduced to about 2 tablespoons, 5 to 7 minutes. Add the coconut oil, stir until well combined, and remove from the heat. Whisk in the cocoa powder, salt, cinnamon, cardamom, and zest. Then add the almonds and stir to coat them. Spread the mixture onto the prepared baking sheet.
3. Bake the nuts for 10 to 12 minutes, stirring halfway through, until toasted. Allow to cool.
4. Store the nuts in an airtight container at room temperature for up to 2 weeks. Make the Banana N'ice Cream: 5. Put the frozen bananas in a food processor and pulse. Scrape down the sides, then pulse once more. Continue to do this for several minutes until the texture resembles ice cream.

Serve immediately with the cooled nuts.

Per Serving:calories: 199 / fat: 14g / protein: 6g / carbs: 16g / sugars: 7g / fiber: 4g / sodium: 195mg

Crustless Peanut Butter Cheesecake

Prep time: 10 minutes / Cook time: 10 minutes / Serves 2

- 4 ounces (113 g) cream cheese, softened
- 2 tablespoons confectioners' erythritol
- 1 tablespoon all-natural, no-sugar-added peanut butter
- ½ teaspoon vanilla extract
- 1 large egg, whisked

1. In a medium bowl, mix cream cheese and erythritol until smooth. Add peanut butter and vanilla, mixing until smooth. Add egg and stir just until combined.
2. Spoon mixture into an ungreased springform pan and place into air fryer basket. Adjust the temperature to 300ºF (149ºC) and bake for 10 minutes. Edges will be firm, but center will be mostly set with only a small amount of jiggle when done.
3. Let pan cool at room temperature 30 minutes, cover with plastic wrap, then place into refrigerator at least 2 hours. Serve chilled.

Per Serving:calorie: 363 / fat: 32g / protein: 12g / carbs: 5g / sugars: 2g / fiber: 0g / sodium: 317mg

Oatmeal Chippers

Prep time: 10 minutes / Cook time: 11 minutes / Makes 20 chippers

- 3–3½ tablespoons almond butter (or tigernut butter, for nut-free)
- ¼ cup pure maple syrup
- ¼ cup brown rice syrup
- 2 teaspoons pure vanilla extract
- 1⅓ cups oat flour
- 1 cup + 2 tablespoons rolled oats
- 1½ teaspoons baking powder
- ½ teaspoon cinnamon
- ¼ teaspoon sea salt
- 2–3 tablespoons sugar-free nondairy chocolate chips

1. Preheat the oven to 350°F. Line a baking sheet with parchment paper.
2. In the bowl of a mixer, combine the almond butter, maple syrup, brown rice syrup, and vanilla. Using the paddle attachment, mix on low speed for a couple of minutes, until creamy. Turn off the mixer and add the flour, oats, baking powder, cinnamon, salt, and chocolate chips. Mix on low speed until incorporated. Place 1½-tablespoon mounds on the prepared baking sheet, spacing them 1" to 2" apart,

and flatten slightly. Bake for 11 minutes, or until just set to the touch. Remove from the oven, let cool on the pan for just a minute, and then transfer the cookies to a cooling rack.

Per Serving:calorie: 90 / fat: 2g / protein: 2g / carbs: 16g / sugars: 4g / fiber: 2g / sodium: 75mg

Cinnamon Spiced Baked Apples

Prep time: 10 minutes / Cook time: 15 minutes / Serves 4

- 2 apples, peeled, cored, and chopped
- 2 tablespoons pure maple syrup
- ½ teaspoon cinnamon
- ½ teaspoon ground ginger
- ¼ cup chopped pecans

1. Preheat the oven to 350°F.
2. In a bowl, mix the apples, syrup, cinnamon, and ginger. Pour the mixture into a 9-inch square baking dish. Sprinkle the pecans over the top.
3. Bake until the apples are tender, about 15 minutes.

Per Serving:calories: 122 / fat: 5g / protein: 1g / carbs: 20g / sugars: 14g / fiber: 3g / sodium: 2mg

Goat Cheese–Stuffed Pears

Prep time: 6 minutes / Cook time: 2 minutes / Serves 4

- 2 ounces goat cheese, at room temperature
- 2 teaspoons pure maple syrup
- 2 ripe, firm pears, halved lengthwise and cored
- 2 tablespoons chopped pistachios, toasted

1. Pour 1 cup of water into the electric pressure cooker and insert a wire rack or trivet.
2. In a small bowl, combine the goat cheese and maple syrup.
3. Spoon the goat cheese mixture into the cored pear halves. Place the pears on the rack inside the pot, cut-side up.
4. Close and lock the lid of the pressure cooker. Set the valve to sealing.
5. Cook on high pressure for 2 minutes.
6. When the cooking is complete, hit Cancel and quick release the pressure.
7. Once the pin drops, unlock and remove the lid.
8. Using tongs, carefully transfer the pears to serving plates.
9. Sprinkle with pistachios and serve immediately.

Per Serving:½ pear: calories: 120 / fat: 5g / protein: 4g / carbs: 17g / sugars: 11g / fiber: 3g / sodium: 54mg

5-Ingredient Chunky Cherry and Peanut Butter Cookies

Prep time: 5 minutes / Cook time: 10 to 12 minutes / Makes 12 cookies

- 1 cup (240 g) all-natural peanut butter

- ¼ cup (60 ml) pure maple syrup
- 1 large egg, beaten
- 1 cup (80 g) gluten-free rolled or quick oats
- ½ cup (80 g) dried cherries

1. Preheat the oven to 350°F (177°C). Line a large baking sheet with parchment paper.
2. In a large bowl, whisk together the peanut butter, maple syrup, and egg. Add the oats and cherries, and mix until the ingredients are combined.
3. Chill the dough for 10 to 15 minutes.
4. Use a cookie scoop to scoop balls of the dough onto the prepared baking sheet.
5. Using a fork, gently flatten the dough balls into your desired shape (the cookies will not change shape much during baking). Bake the cookies for 10 to 12 minutes, until they are lightly golden on top.
6. Remove the cookies from the oven and let them cool for 5 minutes before transferring them to a wire rack.

Per Serving:calorie: 198 / fat: 12g / protein: 7g / carbs: 19g / sugars: 11g / fiber: 3g / sodium: 13mg

Tapioca Berry Parfaits

Prep time: 10 minutes / Cook time: 6 minutes / Serves 4

- 2 cups unsweetened almond milk
- ½ cup small pearl tapioca, rinsed and still wet
- 1 teaspoon almond extract
- 1 tablespoon pure maple syrup
- 2 cups berries
- ¼ cup slivered almonds

1. Pour the almond milk into the electric pressure cooker. Stir in the tapioca and almond extract.
2. Close and lock the lid of the pressure cooker. Set the valve to sealing.
3. Cook on High pressure for 6 minutes.
4. When the cooking is complete, hit Cancel. Allow the pressure to release naturally for 10 minutes, then quick release any remaining pressure.
5. Once the pin drops, unlock and remove the lid. Remove the pot to a cooling rack.
6. Stir in the maple syrup and let the mixture cool for about an hour.
7. In small glasses, create several layers of tapioca, berries, and almonds. Refrigerate for 1 hour.
8. Serve chilled.

Per Serving:½ cup: calories: 174 / fat: 5g / protein: 3g / carbs: 32g / sugars: 11g / fiber: 3g / sodium: 77mg

Mixed-Berry Cream Tart

Prep time: 20 minutes / Cook time: 0 minutes / Serves 8

- 2 cups sliced fresh strawberries
- ½ cup boiling water
- 1 box (4-serving size) sugar-free strawberry gelatin

- 3 pouches (1½ ounces each) roasted almond crunchy granola bars (from 8. 9-oz box)
- 1 package (8 ounces) fat-free cream cheese
- ¼ cup sugar
- ¼ teaspoon almond extract
- 1 cup fresh blueberries
- 1 cup fresh raspberries
- Fat-free whipped topping, if desired

1. In small bowl, crush 1 cup of the strawberries with pastry blender or fork. Reserve remaining 1 cup strawberries.
2. In medium bowl, pour boiling water over gelatin; stir about 2 minutes or until gelatin is completely dissolved. Stir crushed strawberries into gelatin. Refrigerate 20 minutes.
3. Meanwhile, leaving granola bars in pouches, crush granola bars with rolling pin. Sprinkle crushed granola in bottom of 9-inch ungreased glass pie plate, pushing crumbs up side of plate to make crust.
4. In small bowl, beat cream cheese, sugar and almond extract with electric mixer on medium-high speed until smooth. Drop by spoonfuls over crushed granola; gently spread to cover bottom of crust.
5. Gently fold blueberries, raspberries and remaining 1 cup strawberries into gelatin mixture. Spoon over cream cheese mixture. Refrigerate about 3 hours or until firm. Serve topped with whipped topping.

Per Serving:calorie: 170 / fat: 3g / protein: 8g / carbs: 27g / sugars: 17g / fiber: 3g / sodium: 340mg

Watermelon-Lime Granita

Prep time: 15 minutes / Cook time: 0 minutes / Serves 10

- 1 pound seedless watermelon flesh, cut into 1-inch chunks
- 2 tablespoons agave syrup
- 2 tablespoons freshly squeezed lime juice

1. Line a baking sheet with parchment paper. Spread the watermelon chunks in a single layer on the sheet and freeze for at least 20 minutes.
2. Once the chunks are frozen, transfer them to a blender with the agave syrup and lime juice. Blend until liquefied and pour the mixture into a 9-by-13-inch shallow baking dish. Return to the freezer and freeze for 2 hours.
3. Every 30 minutes or so, take a fork and scrape the crystals into a slush consistency. Keep in the freezer for up to 1 month.

Per Serving:calories: 23 / fat: 0g / protein: 0g / carbs: 6g / sugars: 5g / fiber: 0g / sodium: 1mg

Pineapple-Peanut Nice Cream

Prep time: 10 minutes / Cook time: 0 minutes / Serves 6

- 2 cups frozen pineapple
- 1 cup peanut butter (no added sugar, salt, or fat)
- ½ cup unsweetened almond milk

1. In a blender or food processor, combine the frozen pineapple and peanut butter and process.
2. Add the almond milk, and blend until smooth. The end result should be a smooth paste.

Per Serving:calories: 143 / fat: 3g / protein: 10g / carbs: 15g / sugars: 7g / fiber: 3g / sodium: 22mg

Lemon Dessert Shots

Prep time: 30 minutes / Cook time: 0 minutes / Serves 12

- 10 gingersnap cookies
- 2 ounces ⅓-less-fat cream cheese (Neufchâtel), softened
- ½ cup marshmallow crème (from 7 ounces jar)
- 1 container (6 ounces) fat-free Greek honey vanilla yogurt
- ½ cup lemon curd (from 10 ounces jar)
- 36 fresh raspberries
- ½ cup frozen (thawed) lite whipped topping

1. In 1-quart resealable food-storage plastic bag, place cookies; seal bag. Crush with rolling pin or meat mallet; place in small bowl.
2. In medium bowl, beat cream cheese and marshmallow crème with electric mixer on low speed until smooth. Beat in yogurt until blended. Place mixture in 1-quart resealable food-storage plastic bag; seal bag. In 1-pint resealable food-storage plastic bag, place lemon curd; seal bag. Cut 1/8-inch opening diagonally across bottom corner of each bag.
3. In bottom of each of 12 (2-oz) shot glasses, place 1 raspberry. For each glass, pipe about 2 teaspoons yogurt mixture over raspberry. Pipe 1/4-inch ring of lemon curd around edge of glass; sprinkle with about 1 teaspoon cookies. Repeat. 4 Garnish each dessert shot with dollop of about 2 teaspoons whipped topping and 1 raspberry. Place in 9-inch square pan. Refrigerate 30 minutes or until chilled but no longer than 3 hours.

Per Serving:calorie: 110 / fat: 3g / protein: 2g / carbs: 18g / sugars: 14g / fiber: 0g / sodium: 70mg

Cream Cheese Shortbread Cookies

Prep time: 30 minutes / Cook time: 20 minutes / Makes 12 cookies

- ¼ cup coconut oil, melted
- 2 ounces (57 g) cream cheese, softened
- ½ cup granular erythritol

- 1 large egg, whisked
- 2 cups blanched finely ground almond flour
- 1 teaspoon almond extract

1. Combine all ingredients in a large bowl to form a firm ball.
2. Place dough on a sheet of plastic wrap and roll into a 12-inch-long log shape. Roll log in plastic wrap and place in refrigerator 30 minutes to chill.
3. Remove log from plastic and slice into twelve equal cookies. Cut two sheets of parchment paper to fit air fryer basket. Place six cookies on each ungreased sheet. Place one sheet with cookies into air fryer basket. Adjust the temperature to 320°F (160°C) and bake for 10 minutes, turning cookies halfway through cooking. They will be lightly golden when done. Repeat with remaining cookies.
4. Let cool 15 minutes before serving to avoid crumbling.

Per Serving:1 cookie: calories: 154 / fat: 14g / protein: 4g / carbs: 4g / net carbs: 2g / fiber: 2g

Orange Praline with Yogurt

Prep time: 10 minutes / Cook time: 10 minutes / Serves 6

- 3 tablespoons sugar
- 4 teaspoons water
- ⅓ cup slivered almonds, toasted
- ½ teaspoon ground cinnamon
- ⅛ teaspoon ground cloves
- 1 tablespoon orange zest (optional)
- Pinch kosher salt
- 3 cups plain Greek yogurt

1. Preheat the oven to 375°F. Line a baking sheet with parchment paper.
2. In a small saucepan, stir together the sugar and water and cook over high heat until light golden-brown in color, 3 to 4 minutes. Do not stir, but instead gently swirl to help the sugar dissolve. Add the almonds and cook for 1 minute. The goal is to coat the almonds with the heated sugar (think caramel here) without burning. Pour the mixture onto the prepared baking sheet and set aside to cool for about 5 minutes.
3. Meanwhile, in a medium bowl, stir together the cinnamon, cloves, orange zest (if using), and salt.
4. Break the praline into smaller pieces and toss them in the spices.
5. Evenly divide the yogurt among six bowls and serve topped with the spiced praline. Store the praline in a sealed container at room temperature for up to 2 weeks.

Per Serving:calories: 126 / fat: 3g / protein: 8g / carbs: 16g / sugars: 15g / fiber: 1g / sodium: 250mg

Chocolate Baked Bananas

Prep time: 10 minutes / Cook time: 8 to 10 minutes / Serves 5

- 4–5 large ripe bananas, sliced lengthwise
- 2 tablespoons coconut nectar or pure maple syrup
- 1 tablespoon cocoa powder
- Couple pinches sea salt
- 2 tablespoons nondairy chocolate chips (for finishing)
- 1 tablespoon chopped pecans, walnuts, almonds, or pumpkin seeds (for finishing)

1. Line a baking sheet with parchment paper and preheat oven to 450°F. Place bananas on the parchment. In a bowl, mix the coconut nectar or maple syrup with the cocoa powder and salt. Stir well to fully combine. Drizzle the chocolate mixture over the bananas. Bake for 8 to 10 minutes, until bananas are softened and caramelized. Sprinkle on chocolate chips and nuts, and serve.

Per Serving:calorie: 146 / fat: 3g / protein: 2g / carbs: 34g / sugars: 18g / fiber: 4g / sodium: 119mg

Pumpkin Cheesecake Smoothie

Prep time: 10 minutes / Cook time: 0 minutes / Serves 1

- 2 tablespoons cream cheese, at room temperature
- ½ cup canned pumpkin purée (not pumpkin pie mix)
- 1 cup almond milk
- 1 teaspoon pumpkin pie spice
- ½ cup crushed ice

1. In a blender, combine all of the ingredients. Blend until smooth.

Per Serving:calories: 230 / fat: 11g / protein: 11g / carbs: 25g / sugars: 16g / fiber: 4g / sodium: 216mg

Superfood Brownie Bites

Prep time: 15 minutes / Cook time: 0 minutes / Makes 30

- 1 cup raw nuts (walnuts, pecans, or cashews)
- ½ cup hulled hemp seeds
- ⅓ cup raw pepitas
- ½ cup raw cacao powder
- 1 cup pitted dates
- 2 tablespoons coconut oil
- 1 teaspoon vanilla extract

1. Line a baking sheet with parchment paper.
2. Place the nuts, hemp seeds, and pepitas in a food processor and pulse until the ingredients are a meal consistency. Add the cacao powder, dates, coconut oil, and vanilla extract and pulse until the mixture holds together if you pinch it with your fingers. The dough should ball up and appear glossy, and not be too sticky and wet. If it doesn't stick together enough to form a dough consistency, add water in drops until the correct consistency is reached. Be careful not to add too much liquid. If you do, add more cacao to balance the texture.
3. Scoop out the brownie bite mixture in 1-tablespoon amounts and roll the mixture into balls. Set the balls on the baking sheet and then chill them in the refrigerator for at least 10 minutes to hold their shape.
4. Transfer the balls to a container with a lid and store in the refrigerator until ready to eat. You could eat these immediately, but they are more likely to crumble.
5. Store brownies in an airtight container in the refrigerator for 5 to 7 days.

Per Serving:calories: 145 / fat: 11g / protein: 4g / carbs: 11g / sugars: 7g / fiber: 3g / sodium: 2mg

Sponge Cake

Prep time: 15 minutes / Cook time: 1 hour / Serves 12

- 1 cup fresh berries, rinsed
- 2 tablespoons balsamic vinegar
- 2 tablespoons agave nectar
- 4 large eggs, separated
- ¼ cup granulated sugar substitute (such as stevia)
- ½ cup hot water
- 1½ teaspoons vanilla extract
- 1½ cups almond flour, sifted
- ¼ teaspoon salt
- ¼ teaspoon baking powder

1. Preheat the oven to 325 degrees.
2. In a medium bowl, combine the berries with the balsamic vinegar and agave nectar. Mix well to combine; cover, and set aside to steep.
3. In another medium bowl, beat the egg yolks and sugar substitute until thick and lemon-colored. Add the hot water and vanilla, and continue beating for 3 more minutes.
4. In a large bowl, combine the flour, salt, and baking powder; add to the egg yolk mixture.
5. In a small bowl, beat the egg whites until stiff and fold into the egg yolk mixture. Spoon the batter into an ungreased 9-inch tube pan, and bake at 325 degrees for 50–60 minutes or until a toothpick inserted comes out clean.
6. Remove the cake from the oven, and invert it onto a plate. Allow the cake to sit inverted in its pan for at least 1 hour. Remove the pan and let the cake cool completely. Garnish with fresh berry mixture.

Per Serving:calories: 112 / fat: 8g / protein: 5g / carbs: 7g / sugars: 4g / fiber: 2g / sodium: 76mg

Chapter 10 Stews and Soups

Easy Southern Brunswick Stew

Prep time: 20 minutes / Cook time: 8 minutes / Serves 12

- 2 pounds pork butt, visible fat removed
- 17-ounce can white corn
- 1¼ cups ketchup
- 2 cups diced, cooked potatoes
- 10-ounce package frozen peas
- 2 10¾-ounce cans reduced-sodium tomato soup
- Hot sauce to taste, optional

1. Place pork in the Instant Pot and secure the lid.
2. Press the Slow Cook setting and cook on low 6–8 hours.
3. When cook time is over, remove the meat from the bone and shred, removing and discarding all visible fat.
4. Combine all the meat and remaining ingredients (except the hot sauce) in the inner pot of the Instant Pot.
5. Secure the lid once more and cook in Slow Cook mode on low for 30 minutes more. Add hot sauce if you wish.

Per Serving:calories: 213 / fat: 7g / protein: 13g / carbs: 27g / sugars: 9g / fiber: 3g / sodium: 584mg

Egg Drop Soup

Prep time: 10 minutes / Cook time: 15 minutes / Serves 4

- 3½ cups low-sodium vegetable broth, divided
- 1 teaspoon grated fresh ginger (optional)
- 2 garlic cloves, minced
- 3 teaspoons low-sodium soy sauce or tamari
- 1 tablespoon cornstarch
- 2 large eggs, lightly beaten
- 2 scallions, both white and green parts, thinly sliced

1. In a large saucepan, bring 3 cups plus 6 tablespoons of vegetable broth and the ginger (if using), garlic, and tamari to a boil over medium-high heat.
2. In a small bowl, make a slurry by combining the cornstarch and the remaining 2 tablespoons of broth. Stir until dissolved. Slowly add the cornstarch mixture to the rest of the heated soup, stirring until thickened, 2 to 3 minutes.
3. Reduce the heat to low and simmer. While stirring the soup, pour the eggs in slowly. Turn off the heat, add the scallions, and serve.
4. Store the cooled soup in an airtight container in the refrigerator for up to 3 days.

Per Serving:calories: 82 / fat: 3g / protein: 4g / carbs: 11g

/ *sugars: 6g / fiber: 1g / sodium: 248mg*

Roasted Tomato and Sweet Potato Soup

Prep time: 10 minutes / Cook time: 40 to 50 minutes / Serves 4

- 1½ cups onions, finely chopped
- 2 cups cubed red or yellow potatoes (not russet)
- 2 cups cubed sweet potatoes (can use frozen)
- 3–4 large cloves garlic, minced
- 1¼ teaspoons sea salt
- 1½ cups peeled, quartered onion (roughly 1 large onion)
- 4 cups cubed sweet potato (roughly 1–1¼ pounds before peeling)
- 4 cups (about 1½ pounds) quartered Roma or other tomatoes, juices squeezed out
- 1½ teaspoons dried basil
- 1½ teaspoons dried oregano
- 1 tablespoon balsamic vinegar
- 1 teaspoon blackstrap molasses
- Freshly ground black pepper to taste
- 1⅛ teaspoons sea salt
- 2¼–2½ cups water
- ¼ cup chopped fresh basil (optional)

1. Preheat the oven to 450°F.
2. In a large baking dish, combine the onion, sweet potato, tomatoes, basil, oregano, vinegar, molasses, pepper, and 1 teaspoon of the salt. Cook for 40 to 50 minutes, stirring a couple of times, until the sweet potatoes are softened and the mixture is becoming caramelized. Transfer the vegetables and any juices they've released in the pan to a medium soup pot, add 2¼ cups of the water and the remaining ⅛ teaspoon salt, and use an immersion blender to puree. (Alternatively, you can transfer everything to a blender to puree.) Blend to the desired smoothness, using the additional ¼ cup water if needed. Stir in fresh basil, if using, and serve.

Per Serving:calorie: 152 / fat: 0g / protein: 4g / carbs: 35g / sugars: 14g / fiber: 5g / sodium: 648mg

Spanish Black Bean Soup

Prep time: 5 minutes / Cook time: 1 hour 10 minutes / Serves 6

- 1½ cups plus 2 teaspoons low-sodium chicken broth, divided
- 1 teaspoon extra-virgin olive oil
- 3 garlic cloves, minced

- 1 yellow onion, minced
- 1 teaspoon minced fresh oregano
- 1 teaspoon cumin
- 1 teaspoon chili powder or ½ teaspoon cayenne pepper
- 1 red bell pepper, chopped
- 1 carrot, coarsely chopped
- 3 cups cooked black beans
- ½ cup dry red wine

1. In a large pot, heat 2 teaspoons of the chicken broth and the olive oil. Add the garlic and onion, and sauté for 3 minutes. Add the oregano, cumin, and chili powder; stir for another minute. Add the red pepper and carrot.
2. Puree 1½ cups of the black beans in a blender or food processor. Add the pureed beans, the remaining 1½ cups of whole black beans, the remaining 1½ cups of chicken broth, and the red wine to the stockpot. Simmer 1 hour.
3. Taste before serving; add additional spices if you like.

Per Serving:*calories: 160 / fat: 3g / protein: 9g / carbs: 25g / sugars: 1g / fiber: 8g / sodium: 48mg*

Lentil Stew

Prep time: 10 minutes / Cook time: 30 minutes / Serves 2

- ½ cup dry lentils, picked through, debris removed, rinsed and drained
- 2½ cups water
- 1 bay leaf
- 2 teaspoons dried tarragon
- 2 teaspoons dried thyme
- 2 garlic cloves, minced
- 2 medium carrots, chopped
- 2 medium tomatoes, diced
- 1 celery stalk, chopped
- 1 tablespoon extra-virgin olive oil
- 1 medium onion, diced
- 1 cup frozen spinach
- Salt, to season
- Freshly ground black pepper, to season

1. In a soup pot set over high heat, stir together the lentils, water, bay leaf, tarragon, thyme, and garlic.
2. Add the carrots, tomatoes, and celery. Cover. Bring to a boil. Reduce the heat to low and stir the soup. Simmer for 15 to 20 minutes, covered, or until the lentils are tender.
3. While the vegetables simmer, place a skillet over medium heat. Add the olive oil and onion. Sauté for about 10 minutes, or until browned. Remove the skillet from the heat.
4. When the lentils are tender, remove and discard the bay leaf. Add the cooked onion and the spinach

to the soup. Heat for 5 to 10 minutes more, or until the spinach is cooked.
5. Season with salt and pepper.
6. Enjoy immediately.

Per Serving:*calories: 214 / fat: 7g / protein: 10g / carbs: 31g / sugars: 10g / fiber: 11g / sodium: 871mg*

Fresh Fish Chowder

Prep time: 10 minutes / Cook time: 50 minutes / Serves 6

- 2 tablespoons extra-virgin olive oil
- 1 large garlic clove, minced
- 1 small onion, chopped
- 1 large green bell pepper, chopped
- One 14½-ounce can no-salt-added crushed tomatoes
- 1 tablespoon tomato paste
- ½ teaspoon dried basil
- ½ teaspoon dried oregano
- ¼ cup dry red wine
- ½ teaspoon salt
- ½ teaspoon freshly ground black pepper
- ½ cup uncooked brown rice
- ½ pound fresh halibut, cubed
- 2 tablespoons freshly chopped parsley

1. In a 3-quart saucepan, heat the olive oil over medium-high heat. Add the garlic, onion, and green pepper; sauté for 10 minutes over low heat until the vegetables are just tender.
2. Add the tomatoes, tomato paste, basil, oregano, wine, salt, and pepper. Let simmer for 15 minutes. Add the rice and continue to cook for 15 minutes.
3. Add the halibut, and cook for about 5–7 minutes, until the fish is cooked through. Garnish the stew with chopped parsley and serve.

Per Serving:*calories: 166 / fat: 7g / protein: 8g / carbs: 17g / sugars: 3g / fiber: 3g / sodium: 430mg*

Chicken Vegetable Soup

Prep time: 12 to 25 minutes / Cook time: 4 minutes / Serves 6

- 1 to 2 raw chicken breasts, cubed
- ½ medium onion, chopped
- 4 cloves garlic, minced
- ½ sweet potato, small cubes
- 1 large carrot, peeled and cubed
- 4 stalks celery, chopped, leaves included
- ½ cup frozen corn
- ¼ cup frozen peas
- ¼ cup frozen lima beans
- 1 cup frozen green beans (bite-sized)
- ¼ to ½ cup chopped savoy cabbage
- 14½ ounces can low-sodium petite diced tomatoes
- 3 cups low-sodium chicken bone broth

- ½ teaspoon black pepper
- 1 teaspoon garlic powder
- ¼ cup chopped fresh parsley
- ¼ to ½ teaspoon red pepper flakes

1. Add all of the ingredients, in the order listed, to the inner pot of the Instant Pot.
2. Lock the lid in place, set the vent to sealing, press Manual, and cook at high pressure for 4 minutes.
3. Release the pressure manually as soon as cooking time is finished.

Per Serving:calories: 176 / fat: 3g / protein: 21g / carbs: 18g / sugars: 7g / fiber: 4g / sodium: 169mg

Pasta e Fagioli with Ground Beef

Prep time: 0 minutes / Cook time: 30 minutes / Serves 8

- 2 tablespoons extra-virgin olive oil
- 4 garlic cloves, minced
- 1 yellow onion, diced
- 2 large carrots, diced
- 4 celery stalks, diced
- 1½ pounds 95 percent extra-lean ground beef
- 4 cups low-sodium vegetable broth
- 2 teaspoons Italian seasoning
- ½ teaspoon freshly ground black pepper
- 1¼ cups chickpea-based elbow pasta or whole-wheat elbow pasta
- 1½ cups drained cooked kidney beans, or one 15-ounce can kidney beans, rinsed and drained
- One 28-ounce can whole San Marzano tomatoes and their liquid
- 2 tablespoons chopped fresh flat-leaf parsley

1. Select the Sauté setting on the Instant Pot and heat the oil and garlic for 2 minutes, until the garlic is bubbling but not browned. Add the onion, carrots, and celery and sauté for 5 minutes, until the onion begins to soften. Add the beef and sauté, using a wooden spoon or spatula to break up the meat as it cooks, for 5 minutes; it's fine if some streaks of pink remain, the beef does not need to be cooked through.
2. Stir in the broth, Italian seasoning, pepper, and pasta, making sure all of the pasta is submerged in the liquid. Add the beans and stir to mix. Add the tomatoes and their liquid, crushing the tomatoes with your hands as you add them to the pot. Do not stir them in.
3. Secure the lid and set the Pressure Release to Sealing. Press the Cancel button to reset the cooking program, then select the Pressure Cook or Manual setting and set the cooking time for 2 minutes at low pressure. (The pot will take about 15 minutes to come up to pressure before the cooking program begins.)

4. When the cooking program ends, let the pressure release naturally for 10 minutes, then move the Pressure Release to Venting to release any remaining steam. Open the pot and stir the soup to mix all of the ingredients.
5. Ladle the soup into bowls, sprinkle with the parsley, and serve right away.

Per Serving:calories: 278 / fat: 9g / protein: 26g / carbs: 25g / sugars: 4g / fiber: 6g / sodium: 624mg

Nancy's Vegetable Beef Soup

Prep time: 25 minutes / Cook time: 8 hours / Serves 8

- 2 pounds roast, cubed, or 2 pounds stewing meat
- 15 ounces can corn
- 15 ounces can green beans
- 1 pound bag frozen peas
- 40 ounces can no-added-salt stewed tomatoes
- 5 teaspoons salt-free beef bouillon powder
- Tabasco, to taste
- ½ teaspoons salt

1. Combine all ingredients in the Instant Pot. Do not drain vegetables.
2. Add water to fill inner pot only to the fill line.
3. Secure the lid, or use the glass lid and set the Instant Pot on Slow Cook mode, Low for 8 hours, or until meat is tender and vegetables are soft.

Per Serving:calories: 229 / fat: 5g / protein: 23g / carbs: 24g / sugars: 10g / fiber: 6g / sodium: 545mg

Eggplant Stew

Prep time: 5 minutes / Cook time: 1 hour / Serves 2

- 1 tablespoon extra-virgin olive oil
- 1 small Vidalia onion, chopped
- 2 garlic cloves, chopped
- 1 small red bell pepper, chopped
- 1 small eggplant, chopped
- 1 cup black-eyed peas, fresh or frozen
- 1 medium tomato, diced with juice
- 2 teaspoons dried basil
- 2 teaspoons dried oregano
- ⅛ teaspoon salt
- 3 cups water
- 1 tablespoon red wine vinegar

1. To a large saucepan set over medium heat, and the olive oil and onion. Sauté for about 5 minutes.
2. Add the garlic and bell pepper. Sauté for 5 minutes more, or until the vegetables just begin to soften.
3. Add the eggplant, black-eyed peas, tomato, basil, oregano, salt, and water. Increase the heat to high. Bring to a boil. Reduce the heat to medium-low. Simmer for about 1 hour, or until the eggplant is completely cooked and tender.
4. Stir in the red wine vinegar. Cook for 2 minutes

more.

5. Serve immediately and enjoy!

Per Serving:calories: 156 / fat: 5g / protein: 4g / carbs: 26g / sugars: 14g / fiber: 11g / sodium: 176mg

Chicken Brunswick Stew

Prep time: 0 minutes / Cook time: 30 minutes / Serves 6

- 2 tablespoons extra-virgin olive oil
- 2 garlic cloves, chopped
- 1 large yellow onion, diced
- 2 pounds boneless, skinless chicken (breasts, tenders, or thighs), cut into bite-size pieces
- 1 teaspoon dried thyme
- 1 teaspoon smoked paprika
- 1 teaspoon fine sea salt
- ½ teaspoon freshly ground black pepper
- 1 cup low-sodium chicken broth
- 1 tablespoon hot sauce (such as Tabasco or Crystal)
- 1 tablespoon raw apple cider vinegar
- 1½ cups frozen corn
- 1½ cups frozen baby lima beans
- One 14½ ounces can fire-roasted diced tomatoes and their liquid
- 2 tablespoons tomato paste
- Cornbread, for serving

1. Select the Sauté setting on the Instant Pot and heat the oil and garlic for 2 minutes, until the garlic is bubbling but not browned. Add the onion and sauté for 3 minutes, until it begins to soften. Add the chicken and sauté for 3 minutes more, until mostly opaque. The chicken does not have to be cooked through. Add the thyme, paprika, salt, and pepper and sauté for 1 minute more.
2. Stir in the broth, hot sauce, vinegar, corn, and lima beans. Add the diced tomatoes and their liquid in an even layer and dollop the tomato paste on top. Do not stir them in.
3. Secure the lid and set the Pressure Release to Sealing. Press the Cancel button to reset the cooking program, then select the Pressure Cook or Manual setting and set the cooking time for 5 minutes at high pressure. (The pot will take about 15 minutes to come up to pressure before the cooking program begins.)
4. When the cooking program ends, let the pressure release naturally for at least 10 minutes, then move the Pressure Release to Venting to release any remaining steam. Open the pot and stir the stew to mix all of the ingredients.
5. Ladle the stew into bowls and serve hot, with cornbread alongside.

Per Serving:calories: 349 / fat: 7g / protein: 40g / carbs: 17g / sugars: 7g / fiber: 7g / sodium: 535mg

Taco Soup

Prep time: 5 minutes / Cook time: 20 minutes / Serves 4

- Avocado oil cooking spray
- 1 medium red bell pepper, chopped
- ½ cup chopped yellow onion
- 1 pound 93% lean ground beef
- 1 teaspoon ground cumin
- ½ teaspoon salt
- ½ teaspoon chili powder
- ½ teaspoon garlic powder
- 2 cups low-sodium beef broth
- 1 (15-ounce) can no-salt-added diced tomatoes
- 1½ cups frozen corn
- ⅓ cup half-and-half

1. Heat a large stockpot over medium-low heat. When hot, coat the cooking surface with cooking spray. Put the pepper and onion in the pan and cook for 5 minutes.
2. Add the ground beef, cumin, salt, chili powder, and garlic powder. Cook for 5 to 7 minutes, stirring and breaking apart the beef as needed.
3. Add the broth, diced tomatoes with their juices, and corn. Increase the heat to medium-high and simmer for 10 minutes.
4. Remove from the heat and stir in the half-and-half.

Per Serving:calories: 487 / fat: 21g / protein: 39g / carbs: 35g / sugars: 8g / fiber: 5g / sodium: 437mg

Pumpkin Soup

Prep time: 15 minutes / Cook time: 30 minutes / Serves 6

- 2 cups store-bought low-sodium seafood broth, divided
- 1 bunch collard greens, stemmed and cut into ribbons
- 1 tomato, chopped
- 1 garlic clove, minced
- 1 butternut squash or other winter squash, peeled and cut into 1-inch cubes
- 1 teaspoon paprika
- 1 teaspoon dried dill
- 2 (5-ounce) cans boneless, skinless salmon in water, rinsed

1. In a heavy-bottomed large stockpot, bring ½ cup of broth to a simmer over medium heat.
2. Add the collard greens, tomato, and garlic and cook for 5 minutes, or until the greens are wilted and the garlic is softened.
3. Add the squash, paprika, dill, and remaining 1½ cups of broth. Cover and cook for 20 minutes, or until the squash is tender.
4. Add the salmon and cook for 3 minutes, or just enough for the flavors to come together.

Per Serving:calories: 161 / fat: 6g / protein: 24g / carbs: 5g / sugars: 1g / fiber: 1g / sodium: 579mg

Cheeseburger Soup

Prep time: 5 minutes / Cook time: 25 minutes / Serves 4

- Avocado oil cooking spray
- ½ cup diced white onion
- ½ cup diced celery
- ½ cup sliced portobello mushrooms
- 1 pound 93% lean ground beef
- 1 (15-ounce) can no-salt-added diced tomatoes
- 2 cups low-sodium beef broth
- ⅓ cup half-and-half
- ¾ cup shredded sharp Cheddar cheese

1. Heat a large stockpot over medium-low heat. When hot, coat the cooking surface with cooking spray. Put the onion, celery, and mushrooms into the pot. Cook for 7 minutes, stirring occasionally.
2. Add the ground beef and cook for 5 minutes, stirring and breaking apart as needed.
3. Add the diced tomatoes with their juices and the broth. Increase the heat to medium-high and simmer for 10 minutes.
4. Remove the pot from the heat and stir in the half-and-half.
5. Serve topped with the cheese.

Per Serving:calories: 423 / fat: 21g / protein: 39g / carbs: 22g / sugars: 7g / fiber: 3g / sodium: 171mg

Lentil Soup

Prep time: 10 minutes / Cook time: 55 minutes / Serves 8

- 1 large onion, diced
- 1 large carrot, peeled and diced
- 2 stalks celery, diced
- 2 tablespoons extra-virgin olive oil
- 1 pound lentils
- 1½ quarts low-sodium chicken or beef broth
- 2 medium russet or white potatoes, peeled and diced
- 1 tablespoon finely chopped fresh oregano
- 1 teaspoon finely chopped fresh thyme

1. In a stockpot or Dutch oven, sauté the onion, carrot, and celery in the olive oil for 10 minutes. Add the lentils, broth, and potatoes.
2. Continue to cook for 30–45 minutes, adding the oregano and thyme 15 minutes before serving. Soup will keep for 3 days in the refrigerator or can be frozen for 3 months.

Per Serving:calories: 174 / fat: 2g / protein: 8g / carbs: 36g / sugars: 2g / fiber: 3g / sodium: 81mg

Turkey Barley Vegetable Soup

Prep time: 5 minutes / Cook time: 20 minutes / Serves 8

- 2 tablespoons avocado oil
- 1 pound ground turkey
- 4 cups Chicken Bone Broth, low-sodium store-bought chicken broth, or water
- 1 (28-ounce) carton or can diced tomatoes
- 2 tablespoons tomato paste
- 1 (15-ounce) package frozen chopped carrots (about 2½ cups)
- 1 (15-ounce) package frozen peppers and onions (about 2½ cups)
- ⅓ cup dry barley
- 1 teaspoon kosher salt
- ¼ teaspoon freshly ground black pepper
- 2 bay leaves

1. Set the electric pressure cooker to the Sauté/More setting. When the pot is hot, pour in the avocado oil.
2. Add the turkey to the pot and sauté, stirring frequently to break up the meat, for about 7 minutes or until the turkey is no longer pink. Hit Cancel.
3. Add the broth, tomatoes and their juices, and tomato paste. Stir in the carrots, peppers and onions, barley, salt, pepper, and bay leaves.
4. Close and lock the lid of the pressure cooker. Set the valve to sealing.
5. Cook on high pressure for 20 minutes.
6. When the cooking is complete, hit Cancel and allow the pressure to release naturally for 10 minutes, then quick release any remaining pressure.
7. Once the pin drops, unlock and remove the lid. Discard the bay leaves.
8. Spoon into bowls and serve.

Per Serving:calories: 203 / fat: 9g / protein: 15g / carbs: 18g / sugars: 8g / fiber: 6g / sodium: 793mg

Cream of Carrot Soup

Prep time: 5 minutes / Cook time: 15 minutes / Serves 4

- 1 cup plus 2 tablespoons low-sodium chicken broth, divided
- 3 tablespoons finely chopped shallots or onions
- 2 tablespoons flour
- 2 cups fat-free milk, scalded and hot
- 1 teaspoon cinnamon
- 1 cup cooked, pureed carrots
- Freshly ground black pepper

1. In a stockpot, heat 2 tablespoons of the broth over medium heat. Add the shallots and cook until limp. Sprinkle the shallots with the flour and cook 2–3 minutes.
2. Pour in the hot milk and cook until the mixture thickens. Add the remaining ingredients. Bring almost to a boil, stirring often, and cook for approximately 5 minutes. Add pepper to taste.

*Per Serving:*calories: 77 / fat: 1g / protein: 6g / carbs: 12g / sugars: 7g / fiber: 1g / sodium: 89mg

Chock-Full-of-Vegetables Chicken Soup

Prep time: 5 minutes / Cook time: 15 minutes / Serves 2

- 1 tablespoon extra-virgin olive oil
- 8 ounces chicken tenders, cut into bite-size chunks
- 1 small zucchini, finely diced
- 1 cup sliced fresh button mushrooms
- 2 medium carrots, thinly sliced
- 2 celery stalks, thinly sliced
- 1 large shallot, finely chopped
- 1 garlic clove, minced
- 1 tablespoon dried parsley
- 1 teaspoon dried marjoram
- ⅛ teaspoon salt
- 2 plum tomatoes, chopped
- 2 cups reduced-sodium chicken broth
- 1½ cups packed baby spinach

1. In a large saucepan set over medium-high heat, heat olive oil.
2. Add the chicken. Cook for 3 to 4 minutes, stirring occasionally, or until browned. Transfer to a plate. Set aside.
3. To the saucepan, add the zucchini, mushrooms, carrots, celery, shallot, garlic, parsley, marjoram, and salt. Cook for 2 to 3 minutes, stirring frequently, until the vegetables are slightly softened.
4. Add the tomatoes and chicken broth. Increase the heat to high. Bring to a boil, stirring occasionally. Reduce the heat to low. Simmer for 5 minutes, or until the vegetables are tender.
5. Stir in the spinach, cooked chicken, and any accumulated juices on the plate. Cook for about 2 minutes, stirring, until the chicken is heated through.
6. Serve hot and enjoy!

*Per Serving:*calories: 262 / fat: 10g / protein: 32g / carbs: 16g / sugars: 3g / fiber: 6g / sodium: 890mg

Ground Turkey Stew

Prep time: 5 minutes / Cook time: 25 minutes / Serves 5

- 1 tablespoon olive oil
- 1 onion, chopped
- 1 pound ground turkey
- ½ teaspoon garlic powder
- 1 teaspoon chili powder
- ¾ teaspoon cumin
- 2 teaspoons coriander
- 1 teaspoon dried oregano
- ½ teaspoon salt
- 1 green pepper, chopped
- 1 red pepper, chopped
- 1 tomato, chopped
- 1½ cups reduced-sodium tomato sauce
- 1 tablespoon low-sodium soy sauce
- 1 cup water
- 2 handfuls cilantro, chopped
- 15-ounce can reduced-salt black beans

1. Press the Sauté function on the control panel of the Instant Pot.
2. Add the olive oil to the inner pot and let it get hot. Add onion and sauté for a few minutes, or until light golden.
3. Add ground turkey. Break the ground meat using a wooden spoon to avoid formation of lumps. Sauté for a few minutes, until the pink color has faded.
4. Add garlic powder, chili powder, cumin, coriander, dried oregano, and salt. Combine well. Add green pepper, red pepper, and chopped tomato. Combine well.
5. Add tomato sauce, soy sauce, and water; combine well.
6. Close and secure the lid. Click on the Cancel key to cancel the Sauté mode. Make sure the pressure release valve on the lid is in the sealing position.
7. Click on Manual function first and then select high pressure. Click the + button and set the time to 15 minutes.
8. You can either have the steam release naturally (it will take around 20 minutes) or, after 10 minutes, turn the pressure release valve on the lid to venting and release steam. Be careful as the steam is very hot. After the pressure has released completely, open the lid.
9. If the stew is watery, turn on the Sauté function and let it cook for a few more minutes with the lid off.
10. Add cilantro and can of black beans, combine well, and let cook for a few minutes.

*Per Serving:*calories: 209 / fat: 3g / protein: 24g / carbs: 21g / sugars: 8g / fiber: 6g / sodium: 609mg

Italian Vegetable Soup

Prep time: 20 minutes / Cook time: 5 to 9 hours / Serves 6

- 3 small carrots, sliced
- 1 small onion, chopped
- 2 small potatoes, diced
- 2 tablespoons chopped parsley
- 1 garlic clove, minced
- 3 teaspoons sodium-free beef bouillon powder
- 1¼ teaspoons dried basil
- ¼ teaspoon pepper
- 16-ounce can red kidney beans, undrained
- 3 cups water
- 14½-ounce can stewed tomatoes, with juice
- 1 cup diced, extra-lean, lower-sodium cooked ham

1. In the inner pot of the Instant Pot, layer the carrots, onion, potatoes, parsley, garlic, beef bouillon, basil, pepper, and kidney beans. Do not stir. Add water.
2. Secure the lid and cook on the Low Slow Cook mode for 8–9 hours, or on high 4½–5½ hours, until vegetables are tender.
3. Remove the lid and stir in the tomatoes and ham. Secure the lid again and cook on high Slow Cook mode for 10–15 minutes more.

*Per Serving:*calories: 156 / fat: 1g / protein: 9g / carbs: 29g / sugars: 8g / fiber: 5g / sodium: 614mg

Green Ginger Soup

Prep time: 10 minutes / Cook time: 30 minutes / Serves 2

- ½ cup chopped onion
- ½ cup peeled, chopped fennel
- 1 small zucchini, chopped
- ½ cup frozen lima beans
- ¼ cup uncooked brown rice
- 1 bay leaf
- 1 teaspoon dried basil
- ⅛ teaspoon freshly ground black pepper
- 2 cups water
- 1 cup frozen green beans
- ¼ cup fresh parsley, chopped
- 1 (3-inch) piece fresh ginger, peeled, grated, and pressed through a strainer to extract the juice (about 2 to 3 tablespoons)
- Salt, to season
- 2 tablespoons chopped fresh chives

1. In a large pot set over medium-high heat, stir together the onion, fennel, zucchini, lima beans, rice, bay leaf, basil, pepper, and water. Bring to a boil. Reduce the heat to low. Simmer for 15 minutes.
2. Add the green beans. Simmer for about 5 minutes, uncovered, until tender.
3. Stir in the parsley.

4. Remove and discard the bay leaf.
5. In a blender or food processor, purée the soup in batches until smooth, adding water if necessary to thin.
6. Blend in the ginger juice.
7. Season with salt. Garnish with the chives.
8. Serve hot and enjoy immediately!

*Per Serving:*calories: 189 / fat: 2g / protein: 7g / carbs: 39g / sugars: 3g / fiber: 7g / sodium: 338mg

French Market Soup

Prep time: 20 minutes / Cook time: 1 hour / Serves 8

- 2 cups mixed dry beans, washed with stones removed
- 7 cups water
- 1 ham hock, all visible fat removed
- 1 teaspoon salt
- ¼ teaspoon pepper
- 16-ounce can low-sodium tomatoes
- 1 large onion, chopped
- 1 garlic clove, minced
- 1 chile, chopped, or 1 teaspoon chili powder
- ¼ cup lemon juice

1. Combine all ingredients in the inner pot of the Instant Pot.
2. Secure the lid and make sure vent is set to sealing. Using Manual, set the Instant Pot to cook for 60 minutes.
3. When cooking time is over, let the pressure release naturally. When the Instant Pot is ready, unlock the lid, then remove the bone and any hard or fatty pieces. Pull the meat off the bone and chop into small pieces. Add the ham back into the Instant Pot.

*Per Serving:*calories: 191 / fat: 4g / protein: 12g / carbs: 29g / sugars: 5g / fiber: 7g / sodium: 488mg

Chapter 11 Salads

Celery and Apple Salad with Cider Vinaigrette

Prep time: 20 minutes / Cook time: 0 minutes / Serves 4

- Dressing
- 2 tablespoons apple cider or apple juice
- 1 tablespoon cider vinegar
- 2 teaspoons canola oil
- 2 teaspoons finely chopped shallots
- ½ teaspoon Dijon mustard
- ½ teaspoon honey   • ½ teaspoon salt
- Salad
- 2 cups chopped romaine lettuce
- 2 cups diagonally sliced celery
- ½ medium apple, unpeeled, sliced very thin (about 1 cup)
- ⅓ cup sweetened dried cranberries
- 2 tablespoons chopped walnuts
- 2 tablespoons crumbled blue cheese

1. In small bowl, beat all dressing ingredients with whisk until blended; set aside.
2. In medium bowl, place lettuce, celery, apple and cranberries; toss with dressing. To serve, arrange salad on 4 plates. Sprinkle with walnuts and blue cheese. Serve immediately.

Per Serving:calorie: 130 / fat: 6g / protein: 2g / carbs: 17g / sugars: 13g / fiber: 3g / sodium: 410mg

Triple-Berry and Jicama Spinach Salad

Prep time: 30 minutes / Cook time: 0 minutes / Serves 6

- Dressing
- ¼ cup fresh raspberries
- 3 tablespoons hot pepper jelly
- 2 tablespoons canola oil
- 2 tablespoons raspberry vinegar or red wine vinegar
- 2 medium jalapeño chiles, seeded, finely chopped (2 tablespoons)
- 2 teaspoons finely chopped shallot
- ¼ teaspoon salt
- 1 small clove garlic, crushed
- Salad
- 1 bag (6 ounces) fresh baby spinach leaves
- 1 cup bite-size strips (1x¼x¼ inch) peeled jicama
- 1 cup fresh blackberries
- 1 cup fresh raspberries
- 1 cup sliced fresh strawberries

1. In small food processor or blender, combine all dressing ingredients; process until smooth.
2. In large bowl, toss spinach and ¼ cup of the dressing. On 6 serving plates, arrange salad. To

serve, top each salad with jicama, blackberries, raspberries, strawberries and drizzle with scant 1 tablespoon of remaining dressing.

Per Serving:calorie: 120 / fat: 5g / protein: 2g / carbs: 18g / sugars: 9g / fiber: 5g / sodium: 125mg

Raw Corn Salad with Black-Eyed Peas

Prep time: 15 minutes / Cook time: 0 minutes / Serves 8

- 2 ears fresh corn, kernels cut off
- 2 cups cooked black-eyed peas
- 1 green bell pepper, chopped
- ½ red onion, chopped
- 2 celery stalks, finely chopped
- ½ pint cherry tomatoes, halved
- 3 tablespoons white balsamic vinegar
- 2 tablespoons extra-virgin olive oil
- 1 garlic clove, minced
- ¼ teaspoon smoked paprika
- ¼ teaspoon ground cumin
- ¼ teaspoon red pepper flakes

1. In a large salad bowl, combine the corn, black-eyed peas, bell pepper, onion, celery, and tomatoes.
2. In a small bowl, to make the dressing, whisk the vinegar, olive oil, garlic, paprika, cumin, and red pepper flakes together.
3. Pour the dressing over the salad, and toss gently to coat. Serve and enjoy.

Per Serving:calorie: 127 / fat: 4g / protein: 5g / carbs: 19g / sugars: 5g / fiber: 5g / sodium: 16mg

Summer Salad

Prep time: 5 minutes / Cook time: 0 minutes / Serves 4

- For The Salad
- 8 cups mixed greens or preferred lettuce, loosely packed
- 4 cups arugula, loosely packed
- 2 peaches, sliced ½ cup thinly sliced red onion
- ½ cup chopped walnuts or pecans
- ½ cup crumbled feta
- For The Dressing
- 4 teaspoons extra-virgin olive oil
- 4 teaspoons honey

Make The Salad 1. Combine the mixed greens, arugula, peaches, red onion, walnuts, and feta in a large bowl. Divide the salad into four portions.
2. Drizzle the dressing over each individual serving of salad. Make The Dressing 3. In a small bowl, whisk together the olive oil and honey.

Per Serving:calorie: 261 / fat: 19g / protein: 8g / carbs: 20g / sugars: 15g / fiber: 4g / sodium: 184mg

Blueberry and Chicken Salad on a Bed of Greens

Prep time: 10 minutes / Cook time: 0 minutes / Serves 4

- 2 cups chopped cooked chicken
- 1 cup fresh blueberries
- ¼ cup finely chopped almonds
- 1 celery stalk, finely chopped
- ¼ cup finely chopped red onion
- 1 tablespoon chopped fresh basil
- 1 tablespoon chopped fresh cilantro
- ½ cup plain, nonfat Greek yogurt or vegan mayonnaise
- ¼ teaspoon salt
- ¼ teaspoon freshly ground black pepper
- 8 cups salad greens (baby spinach, spicy greens, romaine)

1. In a large mixing bowl, combine the chicken, blueberries, almonds, celery, onion, basil, and cilantro. Toss gently to mix.
2. In a small bowl, combine the yogurt, salt, and pepper. Add to the chicken salad and stir to combine.
3. Arrange 2 cups of salad greens on each of 4 plates and divide the chicken salad among the plates to serve.

Per Serving:calories: 207 / fat: 6g / protein: 28g / carbs: 11g / sugars: 6g / fiber: 3g / sodium: 235mg

Grilled Hearts of Romaine with Buttermilk Dressing

Prep time: 5 minutes / Cook time: 5 minutes / Serves 4

- For The Romaine
- 2 heads romaine lettuce, halved lengthwise
- 2 tablespoons extra-virgin olive oil
- For The Dressing
- ½ cup low-fat buttermilk
- 1 tablespoon extra-virgin olive oil
- 1 garlic clove, pressed
- ¼ bunch fresh chives, thinly chopped
- 1 pinch red pepper flakes

To Make The Romaine 1. Heat a grill pan over medium heat.
2. Brush each lettuce half with the olive oil, and place flat-side down on the grill. Grill for 3 to 5 minutes, or until the lettuce slightly wilts and develops light grill marks.

To Make The Dressing 1. In a small bowl, whisk the buttermilk, olive oil, garlic, chives, and red pepper flakes together.
2. Drizzle 2 tablespoons of dressing over each romaine half, and serve.

Per Serving:calorie: 157 / fat: 11g / protein: 5g / carbs: 12g / sugars: 5g / fiber: 7g / sodium: 84mg

Roasted Asparagus–Berry Salad

Prep time: 10 minutes / Cook time: 18 minutes / Serves 4

- 1 pound fresh asparagus spears
- Cooking spray
- 2 tablespoons chopped pecans
- 1 cup sliced fresh strawberries
- 4 cups mixed salad greens
- ¼ cup fat-free balsamic vinaigrette dressing
- Cracked pepper, if desired

1. Heat oven to 400°F. Line 15x10x1-inch pan with foil; spray with cooking spray. Break off tough ends of asparagus as far down as stalks snap easily. Cut into 1-inch pieces.
2. Place asparagus in single layer in pan; spray with cooking spray. Place pecans in another shallow pan.
3. Bake pecans 5 to 6 minutes or until golden brown, stirring occasionally. Bake asparagus 10 to 12 minutes or until crisp-tender. Cool pecans and asparagus 8 to 10 minutes or until room temperature.
4. In medium bowl, mix asparagus, pecans, strawberries, greens and dressing. Sprinkle with pepper.

Per Serving:calorie: 90 / fat: 3g / protein: 4g / carbs: 11g / sugars: 6g / fiber: 4g / sodium: 180mg

Strawberry-Blueberry-Orange Salad

Prep time: 15 minutes / Cook time: 0 minutes / Serves 8

- ¼ cup fat-free or reduced-fat mayonnaise
- 3 tablespoons sugar
- 1 tablespoon white vinegar
- 2 teaspoons poppy seed
- 2 cups fresh strawberry halves
- 2 cups fresh blueberries
- 1 orange, peeled, chopped
- Sliced almonds, if desired

1. In small bowl, mix mayonnaise, sugar, vinegar and poppy seed with whisk until well blended.
2. In medium bowl, mix strawberries, blueberries and orange. Just before serving, pour dressing over fruit; toss. Sprinkle with almonds.

Per Serving:calorie: 70 / fat: 1g / protein: 0g / carbs: 16g / sugars: 12g / fiber: 2g / sodium: 60mg

Five-Layer Salad

Prep time: 10 minutes / Cook time: 6 minutes / Serves 6

- 1 cup frozen sweet peas
- 1 tablespoon water
- ⅓ cup plain fat-free yogurt
- ¼ cup reduced-fat mayonnaise (do not use salad dressing)

- 1 tablespoon cider vinegar
- 2 teaspoons sugar
- ½ teaspoon salt
- 3 cups coleslaw mix (shredded cabbage and carrots; from 16 ounces bag)
- 1 cup shredded carrots (2 medium)
- 1 cup halved cherry tomatoes

1. In small microwavable bowl, place peas and water. Cover with microwavable plastic wrap, folding back one edge ¼ inch to vent steam. Microwave on High 4 to 6 minutes, stirring after 2 minutes, until tender; drain. Let stand until cool.
2. Meanwhile, in small bowl, mix yogurt, mayonnaise, vinegar, sugar and salt.
3. In 1½- or 2-quart glass bowl, layer coleslaw mix, carrots, tomatoes and peas. Spread mayonnaise mixture over top. Refrigerate 15 minutes. Toss gently before serving.

Per Serving:calorie: 100 / fat: 4g / protein: 3g / carbs: 13g / sugars: 7g / fiber: 3g / sodium: 330mg

Savory Skillet Corn Bread

Prep time: 15 minutes / Cook time: 20 minutes / Serves 8

- Nonstick cooking spray
- 1 cup whole-wheat all-purpose flour
- 1 cup yellow cornmeal
- 1¾ teaspoons baking powder
- ¾ teaspoon baking soda • ½ teaspoon salt
- 1 large zucchini, grated
- 1 cup reduced-fat Cheddar cheese, grated
- ¼ bunch chives, finely chopped
- 1 cup buttermilk • 2 large eggs
- 3 tablespoons canola oil

1. Preheat the oven to 420°F. Lightly spray a cast iron skillet with cooking spray.
2. In a medium bowl, whisk the flour, cornmeal, baking powder, baking soda, and salt together.
3. In a large bowl, gently whisk the zucchini, cheese, chives, buttermilk, eggs, and oil together.
4. Add the dry ingredients to the wet ingredients, and stir until just combined, taking care not to overmix, and pour into the prepared skillet.
5. Transfer the skillet to the oven, and bake for 20 minutes, or until a knife inserted into the center comes out clean. Remove from the oven, and let sit for 10 minutes before serving.

Per Serving:calorie: 239 / fat: 8g / protein: 10g / carbs: 31g / sugars: 3g / fiber: 2g / sodium: 470mg

Sesame Chicken-Almond Slaw

Prep time: 20 minutes / Cook time: 40 minutes / Serves 2

- For the dressing • 1 tablespoon rice vinegar
- 1 teaspoon granulated stevia

- 2 teaspoons extra-virgin olive oil
- 1 teaspoon water • ½ teaspoon sesame oil
- ¼ teaspoon reduced-sodium soy sauce
- Pinch salt
- Pinch freshly ground black pepper
- For the salad
- 8 ounces chicken breast, rinsed and drained
- 4 cups angel hair cabbage
- 1 cup shredded romaine lettuce
- 2 tablespoons sliced scallions
- 2 tablespoons toasted slivered almonds
- 2 teaspoons toasted sesame seeds

1. In a jar with a tight-fitting lid, add the rice vinegar, stevia, olive oil, water, sesame oil, soy sauce, salt, and pepper. Shake well to combine. Set aside. To make the salad:
2. Preheat the oven to 400°F.
3. To a medium baking dish, add the chicken. Place the dish in the preheated oven. Bake for 30 to 40 minutes, or until completely opaque and the temperature registers 165°F on an instant-read thermometer.
4. Remove from the oven. Slice into strips. Set aside.
5. In a large bowl, toss together the cabbage, romaine, scallions, almonds, sesame seeds, and chicken strips. Add the dressing. Toss again to coat the ingredients evenly.
6. Serve immediately.

Per Serving:calorie: 318 / fat: 15g / protein: 31g / carbs: 17g / sugars: 8g / fiber: 6g / sodium: 125mg

Cucumber-Mango Salad

Prep time: 20 minutes / Cook time: 0 minutes / Serves 4

- 1 small cucumber • 1 medium mango
- ¼ teaspoon grated lime peel
- 1 tablespoon lime juice • 1 teaspoon honey
- ¼ teaspoon ground cumin
- Pinch salt • 4 leaves Bibb lettuce

1. Cut cucumber lengthwise in half; scoop out seeds. Chop cucumber (about 1 cup).
2. Score skin of mango lengthwise into fourths with knife; peel skin. Cut peeled mango lengthwise close to both sides of pit. Chop mango into ½-inch cubes.
3. In small bowl, mix lime peel, lime juice, honey, cumin and salt. Stir in cucumber and mango. Place lettuce leaves on serving plates. Spoon mango mixture onto lettuce leaves.

Per Serving:calorie: 50 / fat: 0g / protein: 0g / carbs: 12g / sugars: 9g / fiber: 1g / sodium: 40mg

Curried Chicken Salad

Prep time: 15 minutes / Cook time: 40 minutes / Serves 2

- 4 ounces chicken breast, rinsed and drained

- 1 small apple, peeled, cored, and finely chopped
- 2 tablespoons slivered almonds
- 1 tablespoon dried cranberries
- 2 tablespoons chia seeds
- ¼ cup plain nonfat Greek yogurt
- 1 tablespoon curry powder
- 1½ teaspoons Dijon mustard
- ⅛ teaspoon salt
- ¼ teaspoon freshly ground black pepper
- 4 cups chopped romaine lettuce, divided

1. Preheat the oven to 400°F.
2. To a small baking dish, add the chicken. Place the dish in the preheated oven. Bake for 30 to 40 minutes, or until the chicken is completely opaque and registers 165°F on an instant-read thermometer. Remove from the oven. Chop into cubes. Set aside.
3. In a medium bowl, mix together the chicken, apple, almonds, cranberries, and chia seeds.
4. Add the yogurt, curry powder, mustard, salt, and pepper. Toss to coat.
5. On 2 plates, arrange 2 cups of lettuce on each.
6. Top each with one-half of the curried chicken salad.
7. Serve immediately.

Per Serving:calorie: 240 / fat: 9g / protein: 19g / carbs: 25g / sugars: 14g / fiber: 8g / sodium: 258mg

Three Bean and Basil Salad

Prep time: 10 minutes / Cook time: 0 minutes / Serves 8

- 1 (15 ounces) can low-sodium chickpeas, drained and rinsed
- 1 (15 ounces) can low-sodium kidney beans, drained and rinsed
- 1 (15 ounces) can low-sodium white beans, drained and rinsed
- 1 red bell pepper, seeded and finely chopped
- ¼ cup chopped scallions, both white and green parts
- ¼ cup finely chopped fresh basil
- 3 garlic cloves, minced
- 2 tablespoons extra-virgin olive oil
- 1 tablespoon red wine vinegar
- 1 teaspoon Dijon mustard
- ¼ teaspoon freshly ground black pepper

1. In a large mixing bowl, combine the chickpeas, kidney beans, white beans, bell pepper, scallions, basil, and garlic. Toss gently to combine.
2. In a small bowl, combine the olive oil, vinegar, mustard, and pepper. Toss with the salad.
3. Cover and refrigerate for an hour before serving, to allow the flavors to mix.

Per Serving:Calorie: 193 / fat: 5g / protein: 10g / carbs: 29g / sugars: 3g / fiber: 8g / sodium: 246mg

Romaine Lettuce Salad with Cranberry, Feta, and Beans

Prep time: 10 minutes / Cook time: 0 minutes / Serves 2

- 1 cup chopped fresh green beans
- 6 cups washed and chopped romaine lettuce
- 1 cup sliced radishes
- 2 scallions, sliced
- ¼ cup chopped fresh oregano
- 1 cup canned kidney beans, drained and rinsed
- ½ cup cranberries, fresh or frozen
- ¼ cup crumbled fat-free feta cheese
- 1 tablespoon extra-virgin olive oil
- Salt, to season
- Freshly ground black pepper, to season

1. In a microwave-safe dish, add the green beans and a small amount of water. Microwave on high for about 2 minutes, or until tender.
2. In a large bowl, toss together the romaine lettuce, radishes, scallions, and oregano.
3. Add the green beans, kidney beans, cranberries, feta cheese, and olive oil. Season with salt and pepper. Toss to coat.
4. Evenly divide between 2 plates and enjoy immediately.

Per Serving:calorie: 271 / fat: 9g / protein: 16g / carbs: 36g / sugars: 10g / fiber: 13g / sodium: 573mg

Carrot and Cashew Chicken Salad

Prep time: 20 minutes / Cook time: 25 minutes / Serves 2

- Extra-virgin olive oil cooking spray
- 1 cup carrots rounds
- 1 red bell pepper, thinly sliced
- 1½ teaspoons granulated stevia
- 1 tablespoon extra-virgin olive oil, divided
- ¼ teaspoon salt, divided
- ⅜ teaspoon freshly ground black pepper, divided
- 1 (6-ounce) boneless skinless chicken breast, thinly sliced across the grain
- 2 tablespoons chopped scallions
- 1 tablespoon apple cider vinegar
- 1 cup sugar snap peas
- 4 cups baby spinach
- 4 tablespoons chopped cashews, divided

1. Preheat the oven to 425°F.
2. Coat an 8-by-8-inch baking pan and a rimmed baking sheet with cooking spray.
3. In the prepared baking pan, add the carrots and red bell pepper. Sprinkle with the stevia, 1 teaspoon of olive oil, ⅛ teaspoon of salt, and ⅛ teaspoon of pepper. Toss to coat.
4. Place the pan in the preheated oven. Roast for about 25 minutes, stirring several times, or until tender.
5. About 5 minutes before the vegetables are done,

place the sliced chicken in a medium bowl and drizzle with 1 teaspoon of olive oil. Sprinkle with the scallions. Season with the remaining ⅛ teaspoon of salt and ⅛ teaspoon of pepper. Toss to mix. Arrange in a single layer on the prepared baking sheet.

6. Place the sheet in the preheated oven. Roast for 5 to 7 minutes, turning once, or until cooked through.
7. Remove the pan with the vegetables and the baking sheet from the oven. Cool for about 3 minutes.
8. In a large salad bowl, mix together the apple cider vinegar, the remaining 1 teaspoon of olive oil, the sugar snap peas, and remaining ⅛ teaspoon of pepper. Let stand 5 minutes to blend the flavors.
9. To finish, add the spinach to the bowl with the dressing and peas. Toss to mix well.
10. Evenly divide between 2 serving plates. Top each with half of the roasted carrots, half of the roasted red bell peppers, and half of the cooked chicken.
11. Sprinkle each with about 2 tablespoons of cashews. Serve warm.

Per Serving:calorie: 335 / fat: 17g / protein: 26g / carbs: 21g / sugars: 8g / fiber: 6g / sodium: 422mg

Sofrito Steak Salad

Prep time: 10 minutes / Cook time: 15 minutes / Serves 4

• 4 ounces recaíto cooking base
• 2 (4-ounce) flank steaks
• 8 cups fresh spinach, loosely packed
• ½ cup sliced red onion
• 2 cups diced tomato
• 2 avocados, diced
• 2 cups diced cucumber
• ⅓ cup crumbled feta

1. Heat a large skillet over medium-low heat. When hot, pour in the recaíto cooking base, add the steaks, and cover. Cook for 8 to 12 minutes.
2. Meanwhile, divide the spinach into four portions. Top each portion with one-quarter of the onion, tomato, avocados, and cucumber.
3. Remove the steak from the skillet, and let it rest for about 2 minutes before slicing. Place one-quarter of the steak and feta on top of each portion.

Per Serving:calorie: 314 / fat: 21g / protein: 19g / carbs: 17g / sugars: 5g / fiber: 10g / sodium: 204mg

Shaved Brussels Sprouts and Kale with Poppy Seed Dressing

Prep time: 20 minutes / Cook time: 0 minutes / Serves 4 to 6

• 1 pound Brussels sprouts, shaved
• 1 bunch kale, thinly shredded

• 4 scallions, both white and green parts, thinly sliced
• 4 ounces shredded Romano cheese
• Poppy seed dressing
• Kosher salt
• Freshly ground black pepper

1. In a large bowl, toss together the Brussels sprouts, kale, scallions, and Romano cheese. Add the dressing to the greens and toss to combine. Season with salt and pepper to taste.

Per Serving:calorie: 139 / fat: 7g / protein: 11g / carbs: 11g / sugars: 3g / fiber: 4g / sodium: 357mg

Mediterranean Vegetable Salad

Prep time: 10 minutes / Cook time: 0 minutes / Serves 6

• ⅓ cup tarragon vinegar or white wine vinegar
• 2 tablespoons canola or soybean oil
• 2 tablespoons chopped fresh or 2 teaspoons dried oregano leaves
• ½ teaspoon sugar
• ½ teaspoon salt
• ½ teaspoon ground mustard
• ½ teaspoon pepper
• 2 cloves garlic, finely chopped
• 3 large tomatoes, sliced
• 2 large yellow bell peppers, sliced into thin rings
• 6 ounces fresh spinach leaves (from 10 ounces bag), stems removed (about 1 cup)
• ½ cup crumbled feta cheese (2 ounces)
• Kalamata olives, if desired

1. In small bowl, mix vinegar, oil, oregano, sugar, salt, mustard, pepper and garlic. In glass or plastic container, place tomatoes and bell peppers. Pour vinegar mixture over vegetables. Cover and refrigerate at least 1 hour to blend flavors.
2. Line serving platter with spinach. Drain vegetables; place on spinach. Sprinkle with cheese; garnish with olives.

Per Serving:calorie: 110 / fat: 8g / protein: 3g / carbs: 8g / sugars: 6g / fiber: 1g / sodium: 340mg

Meatless Taco Salad

Prep time: 20 minutes / Cook time: 0 minutes / Serves 2

• ⅓ cup mashed avocado
• ¼ cup plain nonfat Greek yogurt
• 2 tablespoons chopped green bell pepper
• 1 tablespoon chopped scallions
• 1 tablespoon extra-virgin olive oil
• ⅛ teaspoon salt
• ¼ teaspoon chili powder
• ¼ teaspoon freshly ground black pepper
• ½ teaspoon ground cumin
• 3 cups shredded romaine lettuce
• 8 cherry tomatoes, halved

- 1 cup canned kidney beans, rinsed and drained
- ¼ cup sliced black olives
- ½ cup crushed kale chips, divided
- ½ cup shredded nonfat Cheddar cheese, divided

1. In a small bowl, stir together the avocado, yogurt, green bell pepper, scallions, olive oil, salt, chili powder, pepper, and cumin. Set aside.
2. In a large bowl, mix the lettuce, tomatoes, kidney beans, and olives.
3. Evenly divide the lettuce mixture between 2 plates.
4. Top each with half of the avocado mixture.
5. Sprinkle each serving with ¼ cup of kale chips and ¼ cup of Cheddar cheese.
6. Enjoy immediately.

*Per Serving:*calorie: 368 / fat: 21g / protein: 18g / carbs: 30g / sugars: 8g / fiber: 10g / sodium: 613mg

Greek Island Potato Salad

Prep time: 5 minutes / Cook time: 35 minutes / Serves 10

- ⅓ cup extra-virgin olive oil
- 4 garlic cloves, minced
- 2 pounds red potatoes, cut into 1½-inch pieces (leave the skin on if you wish)
- 6 medium carrots, peeled, halved lengthwise, and cut into 1½-inch pieces
- 1 onion, chopped
- 16 ounces artichoke hearts packed in water, drained and cut in half
- ½ cup Kalamata olives, pitted and halved
- ¼ cup lemon juice

1. In a large skillet, heat the olive oil. Add the garlic, and sauté for 30 seconds. Add the potatoes, carrots, and onion; cook over medium heat for 25–30 minutes until vegetables are just tender.
2. Add the artichoke hearts, and cook for 3–5 minutes more. Remove from the heat, and stir in the olives and lemon juice. Season with a dash of salt and pepper. Transfer to a serving bowl, and serve warm.

*Per Serving:*calorie: 178 / fat: 8g / protein: 4g / carbs: 25g / sugars: 4g / fiber: 6g / sodium: 134mg

Chickpea Salad

Prep time: 15 minutes / Cook time: 0 minutes / Serves 4

- ½ cup bottled balsamic vinaigrette
- 1 (15-ounce) can chickpeas, rinsed and drained
- 1 cup cherry tomatoes
- 1 small red onion, quartered and sliced
- 2 large cucumbers, peeled and cut into bite-size pieces
- 1 large zucchini, cut into bite-size pieces
- 1 (10-ounce) package frozen shelled edamame, steamed or microwaved

- Chopped fresh parsley, for garnish

1. Pour the vinaigrette into a large bowl. Add the chickpeas, tomatoes, onion, cucumbers, zucchini, and edamame and toss until all the ingredients are coated.
2. Garnish with chopped parsley.

*Per Serving:*calorie: 188 / fat: 4g / protein: 10g / carbs: 29g / sugars: 11g / fiber: 8g / sodium: 171mg

Strawberry-Spinach Salad

Prep time: 15 minutes / Cook time: 0 minutes / Serves 4

- ½ cup extra-virgin olive oil
- ¼ cup balsamic vinegar
- 1 tablespoon Worcestershire sauce
- 1 (10-ounce) package baby spinach
- 1 medium red onion, quartered and sliced
- 1 cup strawberries, sliced
- 1 (6-ounce) container feta cheese, crumbled
- 4 tablespoons bacon bits, divided
- 1 cup slivered almonds, divided

1. In a large bowl, whisk together the olive oil, balsamic vinegar, and Worcestershire sauce.
2. Add the spinach, onion, strawberries, and feta cheese and mix until all the ingredients are coated.
3. Portion into 4 servings and top each with 1 tablespoon of bacon bits and ¼ cup of slivered almonds.

*Per Serving:*calorie: 417 / fat: 29g / protein: 24g / carbs: 19g / sugars: 7g / fiber: 7g / sodium: 542mg

First-of-the-Season Tomato, Peach, and Strawberry Salad

Prep time: 15 minutes / Cook time: 0 minutes / Serves 6

- 6 cups mixed spring greens
- 4 large ripe plum tomatoes, thinly sliced
- 4 large ripe peaches, pitted and thinly sliced
- 12 ripe strawberries, thinly sliced
- ½ Vidalia onion, thinly sliced
- 2 tablespoons white balsamic vinegar
- 2 tablespoons extra-virgin olive oil
- Freshly ground black pepper

1. Put the greens in a large salad bowl, and layer the tomatoes, peaches, strawberries, and onion on top.
2. Dress with the vinegar and oil, toss together, and season with pepper.

*Per Serving:*calorie: 122 / fat: 5g / protein: 3g / carbs: 19g / sugars: 14g / fiber: 4g / sodium: 20mg

6-Week Meal Plan

	Breakfast	Lunch	Dinner	Snack/Dessert
Monday	Double-Berry Muffins	Fiber-Full Chicken Tostadas	Ahi Tuna Steaks	Classic Crêpes
Tuesday	Mini Breakfast Quiches	Garlic Beef Stroganoff	Vegetable Curry	Dulce de Leche Fillo Cups
Wednesdays	Veggie-Stuffed Omelet	Southwestern Quinoa Salad	Baked Chicken Stuffed with Collard Greens	No-Added-Sugar Orange and Cream Slushy
Thursdays	Potato, Egg and Sausage Frittata	Halibut with Lime and Cilantro	Ginger-Garlic Cod Cooked in Paper	Crustless Peanut Butter Cheesecake
Fridays	Shakshuka	Coconut-Ginger Rice	Shredded Buffalo Chicken	Oatmeal Chippers
Saturdays	Avocado and Goat Cheese Toast	Open-Faced Pulled Pork	Green Beans with Garlic and Onion	Cinnamon Spiced Baked Apples
Sunday	Homemade Turkey Breakfast Sausage	Cobia with Lemon-Caper Sauce	Slow-Roasted Turkey Breast in Beer-Mustard Sauce	Goat Cheese–Stuffed Pears
Monday	Chorizo Mexican Breakfast Pizzas	Salmon Fritters with Zucchini	Lemon Pepper Salmon	Tapioca Berry Parfaits
Tuesday	Lentil, Squash, and Tomato Omelet	Kung Pao Chicken and Zucchini Noodles	Teriyaki Chickpeas	Mixed-Berry Cream Tart
Wednesdays	Baked Berry Coconut Oatmeal	Crab-Filled Mushrooms	Spiced Lamb Stew	Watermelon-Lime Granita
Thursdays	Pumpkin–Peanut Butter Single-Serve Muffins	Chicken Salad	Pico de Gallo Navy Beans	Pineapple-Peanut Nice Cream
Fridays	Cinnamon French Toast	Grilled Rosemary Swordfish	Grilled Scallop Kabobs	Lemon Dessert Shots
Saturdays	Blueberry Cornmeal Muffins	Easy Chicken Cacciatore	Beef Burgundy	Cream Cheese Shortbread Cookies
Sunday	Bacon and Tomato Frittata	Fresh Dill Dip	Garlicky Cabbage and Collard Greens	Orange Praline with Yogurt
Monday	Baked Eggs	Beef Burrito Bowl	Cocoa Coated Almonds	Chocolate Baked Bananas
Tuesday	Hoe Cakes	Peanut Chicken Satay	Lemon-Garlic Mushrooms	Pumpkin Cheesecake Smoothie
Wednesdays	Stovetop Granola	Stewed Green Beans	Baked Salmon with Lemon Sauce	Superfood Brownie Bites
Thursdays	Cheesy Scrambled Eggs	Asparagus with Cashews	Basic Nutritional Values	Sponge Cake
Fridays	Quinoa Breakfast Bake with Pistachios and Plums	Turkey Bolognese with Chickpea Pasta	Fried Zucchini Salad	Southern Boiled Peanuts

Saturdays	Two-Cheese Grits	Salmon Florentine	Steak with Bell Pepper	Cucumber Roll-Ups
Sunday	Potato-Bacon Gratin	Sage and Garlic Vegetable Bake	Snow Peas with Sesame Seeds	No-Bake Coconut and Cashew Energy Bars
Monday	Bunless Breakfast Turkey Burgers	Dandelion Greens with Sweet Onion	Bavarian Beef	Hummus
Tuesday	Sweet Quinoa Cereal	Speedy Chicken Cacciatore	Sautéed Mixed Vegetables	Creamy Cheese Dip
Wednesdays	Carrot Pear Smoothie	Sweet Potato Crisps	Greek Stuffed Tenderloin	Chilled Shrimp
Thursdays	Breakfast Hash	Spicy Citrus Sole	Summer Squash Casserole	Cocoa Coated Almonds
Fridays	Canadian Bacon and Egg Muffin Cups	Herbed Buttermilk Chicken	Homestyle Herb Meatballs	Guacamole with Jicama
Saturdays	Cottage Cheese Almond Pancakes	Baked Garlic Scampi	Roasted Beets, Carrots, and Parsnips	Low-Sugar Blueberry Muffins
Sunday	Wild Mushroom Frittata	Pecan-Crusted Catfish	Herb-Crusted Halibut	Blood Sugar–Friendly Nutty Trail Mix
Monday	Spaghetti Squash Fritters	Italian Bean Burgers	Turkey Stuffed Peppers	Creamy Apple-Cinnamon Quesadilla
Tuesday	Smoked Salmon and Asparagus Quiche Cups	Asparagus with Vinaigrette	Lemony Salmon	Broiled Shrimp with Garlic
Wednesdays	White Bean–Oat Waffles	Gingered-Pork Stir-Fry	Simple Bibimbap	Ginger and Mint Dip with Fruit
Thursdays	Mandarin Orange–Millet Breakfast Bowl	Green Bean and Radish Potato Salad	Smothered Sirloin	Porcupine Meatballs
Fridays	Mexican Breakfast Pepper Rings	Bacon-Wrapped Scallops	Artichokes Parmesan	Hummus
Saturdays	Summer Veggie Scramble	Rice with Spinach and Feta	Spicy Chicken Drumsticks	Monterey Jack Cheese Quiche Squares
Sunday	Baked Berry Coconut Oatmeal	Coconut Curry Rice	Nutmeg Green Beans	Lemony White Bean Puree
Monday	Veggie-Stuffed Omelet	Scallops and Asparagus Skillet	Creole Steak	Baked Scallops
Tuesday	Homemade Turkey Breakfast Sausage	Apple Cinnamon Pork Chops	Balsamic Green Beans and Fennel	Dulce de Leche Fillo Cups
Wednesdays	Bacon and Tomato Frittata	Quinoa Vegetable Skillet	Herb-Roasted Turkey and Vegetables	Oatmeal Chippers
Thursdays	Stovetop Granola	Salmon en Papillote	Fennel and Chickpeas	Cinnamon Spiced Baked Apples
Fridays	Cheesy Scrambled Eggs	Carrots Marsala	Gingered Tofu and Greens	Tapioca Berry Parfaits
Saturdays	Carrot Pear Smoothie	Herbed Cornish Hens	Sun-Dried Tomato Brussels Sprouts	Lemon Dessert Shots
Sunday	Mexican Breakfast Pepper Rings	Low-Sugar Blueberry Muffins	Smoky Pork Tenderloin	Low-Sugar Blueberry Muffins

INDEX

MEASUREMENT CONVERSION CHART

VOLUME EQUIVALENTS(DRY)

US STANDARD	METRIC (APPROXIMATE)
1/8 teaspoon	0.5 mL
1/4 teaspoon	1 mL
1/2 teaspoon	2 mL
3/4 teaspoon	4 mL
1 teaspoon	5 mL
1 tablespoon	15 mL
1/4 cup	59 mL
1/2 cup	118 mL
3/4 cup	177 mL
1 cup	235 mL
2 cups	475 mL
3 cups	700 mL
4 cups	1 L

WEIGHT EQUIVALENTS

US STANDARD	METRIC (APPROXIMATE)
1 ounce	28 g
2 ounces	57 g
5 ounces	142 g
10 ounces	284 g
15 ounces	425 g
16 ounces (1 pound)	455 g
1.5 pounds	680 g
2 pounds	907 g

VOLUME EQUIVALENTS(LIQUID)

US STANDARD	US STANDARD (OUNCES)	METRIC (APPROXIMATE)
2 tablespoons	1 fl.oz.	30 mL
1/4 cup	2 fl.oz.	60 mL
1/2 cup	4 fl.oz.	120 mL
1 cup	8 fl.oz.	240 mL
1 1/2 cup	12 fl.oz.	355 mL
2 cups or 1 pint	16 fl.oz.	475 mL
4 cups or 1 quart	32 fl.oz.	1 L
1 gallon	128 fl.oz.	4 L

TEMPERATURES EQUIVALENTS

FAHRENHEIT(F)	CELSIUS(C) (APPROXIMATE)
225 °F	107 °C
250 °F	120 °C
275 °F	135 °C
300 °F	150 °C
325 °F	160 °C
350 °F	180 °C
375 °F	190 °C
400 °F	205 °C
425 °F	220 °C
450 °F	235 °C
475 °F	245 °C
500 °F	260 °C

The Dirty Dozen and Clean Fifteen

The Environmental Working Group (EWG) is a nonprofit, nonpartisan organization dedicated to protecting human health and the environment Its mission is to empower people to live healthier lives in a healthier environment. This organization publishes an annual list of the twelve kinds of produce, in sequence, that have the highest amount of pesticide residue-the Dirty Dozen-as well as a list of the fifteen kinds ofproduce that have the least amount of pesticide residue-the Clean Fifteen.

THE DIRTY DOZEN

- **The 2016 Dirty Dozen includes the following produce. These are considered among the year's most important produce to buy organic:**

Strawberries	Spinach
Apples	Tomatoes
Nectarines	Bell peppers
Peaches	Cherry tomatoes
Celery	Cucumbers
Grapes	Kale/collard greens
Cherries	Hot peppers

- *The Dirty Dozen list contains two additional itemskale/collard greens and hot peppers-because they tend to contain trace levels of highly hazardous pesticides.*

THE CLEAN FIFTEEN

- **The least critical to buy organically are the Clean Fifteen list. The following are on the 2016 list:**

Avocados	Papayas
Corn	Kiw
Pineapples	Eggplant
Cabbage	Honeydew
Sweet peas	Grapefruit
Onions	Cantaloupe
Asparagus	Cauliflower
Mangos	

- *Some of the sweet corn sold in the United States are made from genetically engineered (GE) seedstock. Buy organic varieties of these crops to avoid GE produce.*

Made in the USA
Monee, IL
25 May 2024

58933283R00059